The Gerstmann's Syndrome Sourcebook

A comprehensive Guide for Patients and Families

Stephanie E. White MAT

Copyright © 2024 Stephanie E. White
All rights reserved.
ISBN: 9798304516976

DEDICATION

To the patients and families navigating the challenges of Gerstmann's Syndrome, your resilience and courage inspire this work.

To the healthcare professionals and researchers who tirelessly seek answers, your dedication brings hope to so many.

And to the readers, may this guide offer clarity, support, and empowerment as you continue your journey.

Contents

1 Introduction 1

2 Understanding Gerstmann's Syndrome 7

3 Causes and Risk Factors 13

4 Signs and Symptoms 19

5 Diagnosing Gerstmann's Syndrome 23

6 Treatment Options 29

7 Living with Gerstmann's Syndrome 35

8 Developmental Gerstmann's Syndrome 41

9 Children and Education 47

10 Navigating Relationships and Communication 53

11 Advances in Research 59

12 Support and Resources 63

13 The History of GS 69

14 Patient Stories 75

15 Frequently Asked Questions 81

16 Looking Forward 87

Appendix A: Medical Glossary 93

Appendix B: Similar Syndromes 99

Appendix C: Resources 103

1 Introduction

Gerstmann's Syndrome is a rare and enigmatic neurological condition that presents unique challenges to patients, families, and caregivers. It is defined by a distinct cluster of symptoms known as the "tetrad": finger agnosia (difficulty recognizing or identifying one's fingers), dysgraphia (difficulty writing), dyscalculia (difficulty performing arithmetic), and left-right disorientation. While these symptoms may seem unrelated at first glance, they share a common neurological origin in the angular gyrus of the parietal lobe. This syndrome, though rare, provides a fascinating glimpse into the interconnected nature of sensory, motor, and cognitive processes within the brain.

For those living with Gerstmann's Syndrome, life can be a daily exercise in problem-solving and adaptation. Tasks that others take for granted—like writing a grocery list, calculating change, or following directions—can become significant hurdles. These challenges can be particularly daunting for children, who may struggle to keep pace with their peers in the classroom, and for adults, who may find their independence diminished after an acquired brain injury. Despite its profound impact on daily living, Gerstmann's Syndrome remains underdiagnosed and often misunderstood, making education and awareness critical.

This sourcebook is designed to serve as a comprehensive guide for individuals affected by Gerstmann's Syndrome, as well as their families, educators, and healthcare providers. Through a combination of scientific insights, practical strategies, and patient stories, this book aims to empower readers with the knowledge and tools needed to navigate life with this condition. Whether you are a parent seeking to support your child, an adult managing the syndrome after a stroke, or a clinician looking for effective treatment strategies, this resource is tailored to meet your needs.

What Makes Gerstmann's Syndrome Unique?

Unlike many neurological conditions, Gerstmann's Syndrome is not defined by a single symptom or physical deficit. Instead, it manifests as a combination of cognitive impairments that disrupt seemingly unrelated tasks. The underlying cause of this syndrome—damage or developmental differences in the angular gyrus—underscores its complexity. This brain region is responsible for integrating sensory input with higher cognitive functions, enabling tasks like identifying fingers, performing calculations, and understanding spatial relationships.

The condition can occur in two forms: developmental and acquired. Developmental Gerstmann's Syndrome (DGS) is observed in children and often manifests as a learning disability, while the acquired form typically arises in adults following a stroke, traumatic brain injury, or tumor. Despite their shared symptomatology, these two forms present distinct challenges and require different approaches to diagnosis and management. This duality highlights the importance of a nuanced understanding of the condition.

The Human Stories Behind the Science

At the heart of Gerstmann's Syndrome are the individuals and families who face its challenges every day. Their experiences are as diverse as the syndrome itself, reflecting the different ways it can impact lives. This book incorporates patient stories to illustrate the real-world implications of the condition and to show how people have found strength, resilience, and innovative solutions.

For instance, Maria, a mother of three, discovered that her youngest child, Ben, had Developmental Gerstmann's Syndrome after years of academic struggles. Ben's inability to grasp basic math concepts, coupled with his frustration over messy handwriting and frequent disorientation, left him feeling isolated in the classroom. Through a combination of occupational therapy, tailored educational strategies, and unwavering family support, Ben found ways to manage his challenges and regain confidence.

Similarly, Alex, a middle-aged professional, experienced Gerstmann's Syndrome after a stroke. Tasks that once felt effortless—writing reports, managing finances, and navigating his surroundings—became sources of frustration. Yet, with the help of a multidisciplinary care team and assistive tools, Alex adapted to his new reality, finding purpose and fulfillment in advocating for others with similar conditions.

These stories remind us that while Gerstmann's Syndrome presents significant challenges, it also reveals the incredible capacity for human resilience and adaptation.

A Comprehensive Approach

One of the primary goals of this book is to provide a well-rounded understanding of Gerstmann's Syndrome, covering everything from its neurological basis to practical coping strategies. The chapters are organized to guide readers through a logical progression of topics, starting with the fundamentals of the condition and moving toward advanced insights and resources. Highlights include:

1. **Understanding the Condition**: An in-depth exploration of the tetrad of symptoms, their neurological origins, and the differences between developmental and acquired forms of the syndrome.
2. **Causes and Risk Factors**: A look at the various causes, including strokes, trauma, and developmental variations, as well as the role of the angular gyrus in brain function.

3. **Signs and Symptoms**: Detailed descriptions of the syndrome's manifestations, with patient stories to illustrate its impact on daily life.

4. **Diagnosis and Treatment**: Insights into clinical assessments, diagnostic tools, and emerging treatments that address both symptoms and underlying causes.

5. **Living with the Syndrome**: Practical advice for managing daily challenges, building support networks, and fostering resilience in patients and families.

Each chapter balances scientific knowledge with actionable strategies, ensuring that readers come away with both a deeper understanding of the condition and the tools to navigate its challenges effectively.

Education, Advocacy, and the Future

Gerstmann's Syndrome is more than a medical condition—it is a call to action for greater awareness, education, and advocacy. For children, early diagnosis and intervention are critical to preventing long-term academic and social difficulties. For adults, access to rehabilitative services and adaptive tools can mean the difference between dependence and independence.

Education is key to breaking down the barriers faced by individuals with Gerstmann's Syndrome. Teachers, parents, and caregivers must work together to create inclusive environments that support learning and growth. Similarly, advocacy groups play a vital role in raising awareness, funding research, and fostering connections within the community.

The future holds promise for individuals with Gerstmann's Syndrome, thanks to ongoing advancements in neuroscience and technology. From neuroimaging techniques that refine diagnosis to innovative therapies like virtual reality training and non-invasive brain stimulation, the possibilities for improving quality of life are expanding. Patient advocacy and collaboration between researchers, clinicians, and families will continue to drive progress, ensuring that no one faces this condition alone.

A Message of Hope

The journey with Gerstmann's Syndrome is not without its challenges, but it is also filled with opportunities for growth, learning, and connection. This book is not just a guide to understanding the condition—it is a celebration of the resilience and determination of those who live with it every day. Through knowledge, support, and perseverance, individuals with Gerstmann's Syndrome can lead fulfilling lives, and families can find strength in the shared journey.

As you begin this book, know that you are not alone. Whether you are seeking answers, looking for practical advice, or simply trying to understand what Gerstmann's Syndrome means for you or your loved one, this resource is here to help. Together, we can illuminate the path forward, fostering a future where everyone affected by Gerstmann's Syndrome has the tools and support they need to thrive.

2 Understanding Gerstmann's Syndrome

What is Gerstmann's Syndrome?

Gerstmann's Syndrome is a rare and complex neurological condition characterized by a unique cluster of cognitive impairments known as the "tetrad." This tetrad includes finger agnosia (difficulty recognizing or identifying one's own fingers), agraphia (difficulty writing), acalculia (difficulty performing arithmetic), and right-left disorientation. These symptoms typically arise from damage to the left angular gyrus, located in the parietal lobe of the brain.

The syndrome is unique in its presentation, as these seemingly unrelated symptoms stem from disruptions in the same brain region. Despite being identified nearly a century ago, Gerstmann's Syndrome remains a topic of fascination and debate in neurology due to its rarity and the occasional overlap with other cognitive and motor impairments.

History and Discovery of the Condition

Gerstmann's Syndrome was first described in 1924 by Josef Gerstmann, an Austrian neurologist. While working with a 52-year-old female patient suffering from cerebral arteriosclerosis, Gerstmann observed a peculiar combination of symptoms affecting her ability to write, count, differentiate fingers, and distinguish right from left. He noted that these impairments occurred independently of her general sensory or motor abilities, suggesting a localized brain lesion.

Over the next several years, Gerstmann refined his observations, identifying the angular gyrus as the likely source of these deficits. By the 1930s, his work had gained recognition, and the term "Gerstmann's Syndrome" was formally adopted to describe this specific tetrad of symptoms. However, the scientific community has long debated whether the syndrome should be considered a distinct clinical entity, as the full tetrad of symptoms is rarely observed in isolation.

A pivotal moment in understanding the syndrome came when neuroimaging technologies, such as CT and MRI, allowed for detailed examination of brain lesions. These advancements confirmed the angular gyrus's critical role, while also revealing that additional brain regions could contribute to the syndrome's manifestations.

Key Features and Symptoms

The hallmark of Gerstmann's Syndrome is its classic tetrad:

- **Finger Agnosia:** Patients struggle to identify, name, or differentiate their fingers, often confusing them with one another. This deficit is bilateral and can extend to recognizing the fingers of others.
- **Agraphia:** Writing abilities are impaired, with patients experiencing difficulty forming letters, words,

or coherent sentences. This deficit often disrupts communication and daily functioning.

- **Acalculia:** The ability to perform basic arithmetic is compromised, even when the patient retains an understanding of numerical concepts. Tasks like addition, subtraction, and multiplication become daunting.
- **Right-Left Disorientation:** Patients find it challenging to distinguish between the right and left sides of their own body or external objects, complicating tasks that require spatial orientation.

While the tetrad defines the syndrome, it is often accompanied by additional symptoms, such as aphasia, constructional apraxia, or visual-spatial deficits, depending on the extent of brain damage. This complexity can make diagnosis challenging.

Who is Affected?

Gerstmann's Syndrome can occur in individuals of all ages, though its causes and manifestations often vary. In adults, the syndrome typically arises from acute brain injuries, such as strokes, traumatic brain injuries, or tumors, that impact the angular gyrus or adjacent regions.

For example, an elderly patient named Maria, recovering from a left-hemisphere stroke, began noticing an unusual set of challenges. She struggled to identify her fingers when asked to point them out and felt frustrated when simple calculations became insurmountable tasks. Despite maintaining her memory and other cognitive functions, these isolated deficits drastically altered her daily life.

In children, Gerstmann's Syndrome is often developmental, emerging as a subtle learning disability rather than an acute condition. For these children, difficulties with writing and math frequently lead to misdiagnosis as a general learning disorder, delaying appropriate interventions.

Patient Stories

Maria's experience is one among many. Another patient, Alex, a middle-aged teacher, was rushed to the hospital after a mild stroke. He noticed he couldn't tell his right hand from his left when trying to put on his shoes and struggled to write the alphabet during therapy sessions. Although Alex regained some abilities with rehabilitation, he continues to experience lingering challenges with arithmetic and spatial orientation.

A younger case involves eight-year-old Lily, whose parents noticed her persistent struggles with writing and identifying her fingers during class activities. Initially dismissed as clumsiness or a lack of focus, Lily was eventually diagnosed with developmental Gerstmann's Syndrome after neuropsychological testing.

Conclusion

Gerstmann's Syndrome is a testament to the intricate interplay between specific brain regions and cognitive functions. While rare, its impact on patients' lives is profound, often challenging their ability to perform basic tasks. Understanding the condition's history, symptoms, and variability is crucial for accurate diagnosis and effective management, offering hope and clarity to those affected.

References

1. Toader C, Covache-Busuioc RA, Rădoi PM, Covlea CA, Popa AA, Dumitrascu DI, et al. Gerstmann Syndrome in an Elderly Patient: A Case Report Presented with a Complete Tetrad of Symptoms. Medicina. 2024;60:1640.

2. Salih AA. Gerstmann Syndrome Case-Control Study: Correlation between Brain Lesions & Functional Disability. Neuropsychol. 2023;27(2):247-252.

3. João RB, Filgueiras RM, Mussi ML, Barros JEF. Transient Gerstmann Syndrome as a Manifestation of Stroke: Case Report and Brief Literature Review. Dement Neuropsychol. 2017;11(2):202-205.

4. Pyrtek S, Badziński A, Adamczyk-Sowa M, Pąchalska M. Does Gerstmann Syndrome Exist? Neuropsychologica. 2020;18(2):259-284.

3 Causes and Risk Factors

Gerstmann's Syndrome is a neurological puzzle, deeply rooted in the complexities of the brain's parietal lobe. The condition's defining tetrad of symptoms—finger agnosia, dysgraphia, dyscalculia, and left-right disorientation—provides a unique window into the interconnectedness of sensory, motor, and cognitive processes. At the heart of this syndrome lies the angular gyrus, a critical region where sensory input meets abstract reasoning, enabling tasks as diverse as identifying fingers and solving mathematical equations.

This chapter delves into the multifaceted causes of Gerstmann's Syndrome, from acute neurological insults like strokes and tumors to the subtler developmental variations observed in children. We explore the interplay between genetic, acquired, and developmental factors, highlighting the condition's diverse presentations. Alongside scientific explanations, we include real patient stories to illustrate the challenges and triumphs of those living with this condition. By understanding the underlying mechanisms and common risk factors, patients, families, and caregivers can better navigate the complexities of Gerstmann's Syndrome, fostering early diagnosis, tailored interventions, and improved outcomes.

Neurological Basis of Gerstmann's Syndrome

At the core of Gerstmann's Syndrome lies a disruption in the intricate network of the brain's dominant hemisphere, typically the left. The hallmark symptoms of this condition—finger agnosia, dysgraphia, dyscalculia, and left-right disorientation—are linked to localized damage in the angular gyrus of the parietal lobe. This area integrates sensory input with cognitive processes, bridging physical sensations and abstract reasoning.

The angular gyrus functions as a crossroads for spatial awareness, numerical understanding, and language. When it is impaired, as in Gerstmann's Syndrome, the effects cascade across multiple cognitive domains. For instance, finger agnosia reflects a breakdown in recognizing spatially encoded sensory inputs, while dyscalculia illustrates the inability to process numerical operations, despite preserved basic numerical understanding.

Underlying Brain Regions Involved

The angular gyrus, nestled at the intersection of the parietal, temporal, and occipital lobes, serves as the epicenter of Gerstmann's Syndrome. Damage here typically arises from strokes, tumors, or trauma. Adjacent structures, including the supramarginal gyrus and intraparietal sulcus, may also contribute to the condition when lesions extend beyond the angular gyrus.

Moreover, studies suggest that disruptions in subcortical white matter, which connects the angular gyrus to other brain areas, exacerbate the syndrome's presentation. This implies that Gerstmann's Syndrome may be as much about disconnection between brain networks as it is about localized damage.

Genetic, Acquired, and Developmental Causes

Gerstmann's Syndrome manifests in various forms, with distinct etiologies depending on the patient's age and circumstances.

1. **Acquired Causes**
   o **Strokes**: Ischemic or hemorrhagic strokes in the left parietal lobe are a leading cause, particularly in older adults.
   o **Trauma**: Brain injuries, such as those from vehicular accidents, can localize damage to the angular gyrus.
   o **Tumors**: Growths like gliomas or hemangiopericytomas exert pressure on the angular gyrus, producing symptoms.
   o **Infections**: Conditions like progressive multifocal leukoencephalopathy or meningitis occasionally involve the parietal lobe.

A particularly striking case involved a 37-year-old man diagnosed with a solitary fibrous tumor in the left parietal lobe. His symptoms included all four features of Gerstmann's Syndrome. Following surgical resection, his symptoms resolved entirely, underscoring the reversible nature of the syndrome in cases with treatable underlying conditions.

2. **Developmental Causes**
Developmental Gerstmann's Syndrome is observed in children without identifiable lesions. These cases are thought to stem from delayed or atypical development of the parietal lobe. Children with this form may exhibit learning difficulties, especially in math and writing, often leading to misdiagnosis as general learning disabilities.

Lily, an eight-year-old diagnosed with developmental Gerstmann's Syndrome, faced persistent struggles in recognizing her fingers during classroom activities. Her parents' perseverance in seeking a diagnosis allowed her to receive targeted interventions, significantly improving her writing and math skills.

3. Genetic Causes

Rare genetic syndromes can occasionally mimic Gerstmann's Syndrome. For example, mutations in the PRNP gene, as seen in Gerstmann-Sträussler-Scheinker Syndrome, lead to progressive neurological decline, including features overlapping with Gerstmann's tetrad.

Common Risk Factors

Several risk factors predispose individuals to Gerstmann's Syndrome, varying across its acquired, developmental, and genetic forms:

- **Age**: Older adults are more vulnerable due to the higher prevalence of strokes, tumors, and neurodegenerative diseases.
- **Medical History**: Conditions such as hypertension, atrial fibrillation, or diabetes increase the risk of strokes that can damage the angular gyrus.
- **Trauma**: Head injuries are a frequent cause of localized brain damage, particularly in younger adults.
- **Neurodegenerative Diseases**: Disorders like Alzheimer's disease occasionally affect the parietal lobe, producing Gerstmann-like symptoms.
- **Exposure to Toxins**: Lead poisoning and chronic alcoholism are associated with parietal lobe dysfunctions.
- **Genetic Predisposition**: A family history of neurological conditions or genetic mutations, like PRNP mutations, can predispose individuals to related syndromes.

Patient Stories

Maria, a retired teacher, experienced profound changes following a minor stroke. At first, her family thought she was simply forgetting small tasks. Over time, her difficulty in distinguishing left from right and her inability to perform basic arithmetic signaled something more serious. An MRI revealed a small lesion in her left angular gyrus. With therapy, Maria regained partial function, though her spatial orientation remained impaired.

In another case, Alex, a 45-year-old mechanic, survived a traumatic brain injury after a car accident. His recovery was complicated by newfound struggles with writing and calculating, both essential to his work. Therapy focused on compensatory strategies, like using calculators and adaptive writing tools, enabling Alex to return to his job.

Conclusion

The causes and risk factors of Gerstmann's Syndrome highlight its complexity, spanning acute injuries, developmental anomalies, and genetic predispositions. Understanding these underlying mechanisms is essential for accurate diagnosis and effective treatment. For patients and families, this knowledge provides hope, emphasizing that with the right interventions, individuals can regain function and improve their quality of life.

References

1. Natteru P, Ramachandran Nair L, Luzardo G, et al. Meningeal Hemangiopericytoma Presenting as Pure Gerstmann Syndrome: A Double Rarity. Cureus. 2021;13(6):e15863.

2. Cao L, Feng H, Huang X, et al. Gerstmann-Sträussler-Scheinker Syndrome Misdiagnosed as Cervical Spondylotic Myelopathy: A Case Report with 5-Year Follow-Up. Medicine. 2021;100:16(e25687).

3. Altabakhi IW, Liang JW. Gerstmann Syndrome. StatPearls. Treasure Island: StatPearls Publishing; 2023.

4. Zeidman LA, Ziller MG, Shevell M. "With a smile through tears": the uprooted career of the man behind Gerstmann syndrome. J Hist Neurosci. 2015;24(2):148-72.

5. João RB, Filgueiras RM, Mussi ML, de Barros JEF. Transient Gerstmann Syndrome as a Manifestation of Stroke: Case Report and Brief Literature Review. Dement Neuropsychol. 2017;11(2):202-205.

4 Signs and Symptoms

Gerstmann's Syndrome, a rare neurological condition, is defined by a characteristic tetrad of symptoms: finger agnosia, dysgraphia, dyscalculia, and left-right disorientation. Each symptom represents a profound challenge, disrupting fundamental aspects of daily life. However, these symptoms often extend beyond the tetrad, with other associated cognitive and perceptual impairments occasionally present. This chapter explores these manifestations through detailed explanations and patient stories, illuminating the lived experiences of those affected by this complex condition.

Finger Agnosia: The Puzzle of Self-Recognition

Finger agnosia, the inability to identify or distinguish between one's own fingers, might seem trivial at first glance, but its impact can be life-altering. Individuals with this condition struggle to name or recognize their fingers, an impairment that often hampers tasks requiring fine motor coordination.

For Maria, a kindergarten teacher, finger agnosia became a significant barrier. Tasks as simple as demonstrating finger-counting exercises for her students turned into moments of confusion. She recounts how she started using color-coded stickers to distinguish her fingers, turning a frustrating limitation into a creative solution. This adaptation became a symbol of her resilience, allowing her to continue teaching while navigating her challenges.

Dysgraphia: The Written Word Disrupted

Dysgraphia, or difficulty in writing, is another defining feature of Gerstmann's Syndrome. Patients may struggle with letter formation, spatial alignment on paper, and overall legibility, making communication through writing a daunting task.

Alex, a journalist, described his journey of adapting to dysgraphia after a stroke left him grappling with the condition. "It was like my hand forgot how to follow instructions," he said. To overcome this, he turned to voice-to-text technology and embraced digital tools for composing articles. Although his handwriting remains impaired, his creativity and voice as a journalist have not been silenced.

Dyscalculia: The Complexity of Numbers

Dyscalculia, characterized by difficulty with mathematical concepts, extends beyond simple arithmetic. Patients often face challenges with numerical reasoning, spatial organization of numbers, and understanding the relationships between quantities.

Liam, a ten-year-old boy diagnosed with developmental Gerstmann's Syndrome, struggled with basic math in school. His parents noted that he had difficulty using money or understanding measurements in cooking. With the help of visual aids and tactile tools, Liam learned alternative ways to approach math problems, enabling him to gain confidence and build foundational skills.

Left-Right Disorientation: A Spatial Conundrum

The inability to distinguish left from right can be deeply

disorienting. This symptom, known as left-right disorientation, affects spatial awareness and body orientation, complicating navigation and daily tasks.

Maggie, a retired librarian, recounted how left-right confusion became a source of anxiety while driving. She often missed turns or hesitated at intersections, unsure of her bearings. After consulting with an occupational therapist, Maggie began using verbal mnemonics and visual markers, which helped her regain a sense of control over her environment.

Other Potential Associated Symptoms

While the primary tetrad of symptoms defines Gerstmann's Syndrome, additional cognitive and perceptual impairments can accompany the condition. These may include constructional apraxia, semantic aphasia, or impairments in visual-spatial processing. Each of these symptoms adds layers of complexity to the patient's experience, requiring comprehensive assessment and tailored support.

One case involved Paul, a 58-year-old mechanic, who experienced severe difficulties with spatial reasoning after a parietal lobe stroke. His ability to assemble and repair machinery was deeply affected. Paul worked closely with a neuropsychologist to develop mental mapping strategies and rebuild his spatial skills, demonstrating the potential for adaptation and recovery even in the face of significant challenges.

Navigating the Intersection of Symptoms

The interplay between the symptoms of Gerstmann's Syndrome creates a unique challenge for patients. Finger agnosia can compound the effects of dysgraphia, while dyscalculia and left-right disorientation may intersect to create difficulties in navigation or understanding spatial relationships. These interdependencies highlight the importance of a holistic approach to diagnosis and treatment, addressing the individual needs of each patient.

Conclusion

The signs and symptoms of Gerstmann's Syndrome paint a picture of resilience in the face of adversity. Each patient's journey is a testament to their adaptability and determination, as they find ways to navigate life's challenges with creativity and strength. By understanding the nuanced experiences of those affected by this syndrome, we can foster empathy, develop better interventions, and support patients in achieving their full potential.

References

1. Patil VC, Kulkarni AR. Gerstmann's Syndrome: A Rare Clinical Condition with a Tetrad of Symptoms. International Journal of Contemporary Medical Research.

2. Morais CPT, Montenegro GR, Rocha IR, et al. Síndrome de Gerstmann. Brazilian Journal of Health Review.

3. Pyrtek S, Badziński A, Adamczyk-Sowa M, Pąchalska M. Does Gerstmann Syndrome Exist? Neuropsychologica.

5 Diagnosing Gerstmann's Syndrome

Clinical Assessment and Tests

Diagnosing Gerstmann's Syndrome requires a comprehensive approach, as its symptoms—finger agnosia, agraphia, acalculia, and right-left disorientation—can overlap with other neurological conditions. The diagnostic process typically begins with a detailed patient history and a thorough clinical evaluation, including neuropsychological tests tailored to each symptom.

For instance, tasks to identify finger agnosia involve asking patients to name, point to, or differentiate their fingers on command. Similarly, writing assessments help uncover agraphia, where patients struggle to form coherent letters or words. Acalculia is evaluated through simple arithmetic tests, while right-left disorientation is tested by asking patients to identify directions on their own or others' bodies. These tasks are crucial to isolating Gerstmann's Syndrome from broader neurological impairments.

Consider Maria, a 68-year-old teacher, who sought medical help after struggling with basic arithmetic and writing. She recounted instances where she mistakenly referred to her left hand as her right. During her assessment, Maria failed tasks requiring her to identify specific fingers, confirming the presence of finger agnosia alongside her other challenges. These evaluations provided the foundation for her diagnosis.

Neurological Imaging (MRI, CT Scans)

Neuroimaging is a cornerstone in confirming Gerstmann's Syndrome, particularly when brain lesions are suspected. Magnetic resonance imaging (MRI) and computed tomography (CT) scans are used to identify damage in the angular gyrus or other critical regions of the left parietal lobe. Advanced imaging techniques, such as diffusion tensor imaging (DTI), can reveal disruptions in white matter tracts connecting the angular gyrus to other parts of the brain.

For example, a 49-year-old magazine editor with Gerstmann's Syndrome underwent an MRI that revealed lesions in the left parieto-occipital region. The images showed decreased connectivity in the superior longitudinal fasciculus, a critical pathway linking sensory and motor integration. This case highlighted how imaging not only confirmed the diagnosis but also provided insights into the neurological basis of the condition.

Differential Diagnosis: Conditions with Similar Symptoms

One of the greatest challenges in diagnosing Gerstmann's Syndrome is distinguishing it from other neurological conditions with overlapping symptoms. Aphasia, constructional apraxia, and visual-spatial deficits can mimic parts of the syndrome, making differential diagnosis essential.

For example, in stroke patients, symptoms like impaired writing or calculation may stem from broader language deficits rather than true agraphia or acalculia. Similarly, right-left disorientation could be part of more extensive spatial neglect. Neuropsychological tests help tease apart these nuances by focusing on the specific tetrad of symptoms unique to Gerstmann's Syndrome.

A particularly notable case involved Alex, a retired engineer who had enjoyed a long and successful career solving complex technical problems. Following a traumatic brain injury sustained in a car accident, Alex began experiencing significant difficulties with writing and performing even simple calculations, tasks that had once been second nature to him. At first, his symptoms were attributed to general cognitive decline associated with aging or the residual effects of the injury. However, as his condition progressed, his family noticed a curious pattern: while Alex retained his verbal fluency and memory, his ability to manage numbers and compose coherent written notes seemed disproportionately impaired.

Specialists initially suspected a mild form of aphasia, but Alex's speech and comprehension remained unaffected. Similarly, while broader spatial neglect was considered a possibility, his ability to navigate his surroundings and interact with objects in space did not align with such a diagnosis. After a series of neuropsychological assessments and imaging studies, his precise pattern of deficits—severe writing and calculation difficulties in the absence of aphasia or spatial neglect—pointed toward Gerstmann's Syndrome. The diagnosis brought clarity, allowing Alex and his family to focus on targeted therapies that improved his quality of life and helped him adapt to the challenges posed by his condition.

Importance of Early and Accurate Diagnosis

Early and accurate diagnosis of Gerstmann's Syndrome is crucial for effective management. Misdiagnosis can delay targeted interventions, exacerbating challenges in daily life. Identifying the syndrome early allows for tailored therapies that address specific deficits, improving patient outcomes.

For children with developmental Gerstmann's Syndrome, timely diagnosis ensures they receive appropriate educational support, preventing academic struggles. For adults with acquired forms, early recognition helps guide rehabilitation, enabling them to adapt to their limitations while maximizing their independence.

Take the story of Lily, an 8-year-old girl whose struggles with math and writing were initially dismissed as a learning disability. A detailed evaluation revealed the classic symptoms of Gerstmann's Syndrome, leading to a tailored intervention plan that significantly improved her academic performance.

Conclusion

Diagnosing Gerstmann's Syndrome requires a careful balance of clinical expertise, neuropsychological testing, and advanced imaging. By isolating its unique symptoms and distinguishing it from similar conditions, healthcare providers can offer patients clarity and direction. Early and accurate diagnosis not only validates the experiences of those affected but also opens the door to interventions that enhance their quality of life.

References

1. Yoon SH, Lee JI, Kang MJ, Lee HI, Pyun SB. Gerstmann Syndrome as a Disconnection Syndrome: A Single Case Diffusion Tensor Imaging Study. Brain Neurorehabil. 2023;16(1):e3.

2. Pyrtek S, Badziński A, Adamczyk-Sowa M, Pąchalska M. Does Gerstmann Syndrome Exist? Neuropsychologica. 2020;18(2):259-284.

3. Orozco Aguirre AL, Marín Valdovino M, Ruíz Santos MA, González Meléndez AM. Secondary Gerstmann Syndrome: A Case Report. Eur Psychiatry. 2022;59(Suppl 1):S478.

4. Arts M. Somatic Comorbidity and Physical Frailty in Elderly with Medically Unexplained Symptoms. Eur Psychiatry. 2022;59(Suppl 1):S478.

6 Treatment Options

Treating Gerstmann's Syndrome requires a nuanced approach, addressing both its underlying causes and the unique challenges posed by its symptoms. As a rare neurological condition, the syndrome demands individualized care to manage the diverse deficits of finger agnosia, dysgraphia, dyscalculia, and right-left disorientation. This chapter explores the various pathways to treatment, from addressing root causes like strokes or trauma to therapies aimed at symptom management.

Medications may play a supportive role, while emerging technologies, such as neuromodulation and deep brain stimulation, hint at future possibilities. Central to effective treatment is a multidisciplinary care team, which combines the expertise of neurologists, therapists, and caregivers to craft personalized strategies. By weaving patient stories with clinical insights, this chapter highlights the importance of a holistic approach to improving quality of life and fostering hope for those affected by Gerstmann's Syndrome.

Addressing Underlying Causes

Treatment for Gerstmann's Syndrome often begins with addressing its root causes, which vary widely from strokes and traumatic brain injuries to tumors and neurodegenerative diseases. In cases where the syndrome arises from acute conditions like a stroke, the priority is immediate medical management to stabilize the patient and prevent further damage. Antiplatelet medications, anticoagulants, and blood pressure management can help mitigate stroke progression and its aftereffects.

For example, Alex, a 54-year-old accountant, experienced sudden difficulty with basic arithmetic and distinguishing his fingers following a mild stroke. Early intervention with blood thinners and rehabilitation focused on regaining his motor and cognitive abilities. Although his symptoms did not completely resolve, early treatment prevented further decline and enabled him to adapt using assistive tools.

When caused by brain tumors, surgical intervention may alleviate symptoms by relieving pressure on the angular gyrus. In one striking case, Maria, a 62-year-old retired teacher with Gerstmann's Syndrome due to a meningioma, underwent tumor resection. Post-surgery, she regained partial functionality in writing and numerical tasks, showcasing the reversibility of some symptoms when the underlying cause is treated effectively.

Therapies for Symptom Management

Managing the symptoms of Gerstmann's Syndrome requires a multidisciplinary approach involving physical, occupational, and cognitive therapies. Each symptom—finger agnosia, dysgraphia, dyscalculia, and right-left disorientation—is addressed through targeted interventions.

- **Finger Agnosia**: Therapists use exercises like finger-pointing games and tactile recognition drills to help patients improve finger differentiation. For instance, children with developmental Gerstmann's Syndrome benefit from repetitive, game-like tasks that make therapy engaging and effective. Eight-year-old Liam, diagnosed with the syndrome, made remarkable progress using finger puppets to learn identification and improve fine motor skills.

- **Dysgraphia**: Writing difficulties are tackled through adaptive tools such as special writing aids or typing programs. Therapists work with patients on fine motor coordination, sometimes using digital apps that guide letter formation.

- **Dyscalculia**: This symptom requires strategies like visual aids, manipulatives, and calculators. In Lily's case, a 12-year-old with developmental Gerstmann's Syndrome, her teacher implemented number-line charts and interactive math games, enabling her to build basic arithmetic skills.

- **Right-Left Disorientation**: Therapies focus on spatial orientation through repetitive drills, including identifying left and right on the patient's own body and on external objects.

Medications and Their Role

While no medications directly treat Gerstmann's Syndrome, pharmacological approaches play a supportive role, particularly when the syndrome stems from other conditions. For example:

- **Neuroprotective Drugs**: In stroke-related cases, medications aimed at preserving brain function, such as edaravone or citicoline, may limit damage.

- **Anti-inflammatory Agents**: In conditions like multiple sclerosis, reducing inflammation in the parietal lobe can mitigate symptoms.

- **Anticonvulsants**: When the syndrome is associated with epilepsy, as in the case of Jared, a 36-year-old with transient Gerstmann's Syndrome, controlling seizures with medications like levetiracetam helped manage episodic symptoms.

Research into advanced interventions, including

neuromodulation techniques like transcranial magnetic stimulation (TMS) and deep brain stimulation (DBS), is ongoing. While these are still experimental, they offer hope for future treatment pathways.

The Importance of a Multidisciplinary Care Team

Effective treatment of Gerstmann's Syndrome hinges on a multidisciplinary team approach, integrating neurologists, neuropsychologists, therapists, and caregivers. Each professional contributes to a comprehensive care plan tailored to the patient's unique needs.

For instance, Maggie, a 45-year-old nurse with Gerstmann's Syndrome following a traumatic brain injury, benefited from a team that included:

- A neurologist managing her recovery from the injury.
- A cognitive therapist helping her relearn basic arithmetic and spatial orientation.
- An occupational therapist guiding her use of adaptive tools at work.
- Supportive caregivers at home, who reinforced therapy exercises and encouraged her progress.

This collaborative approach ensured that Maggie's treatment addressed both her medical and functional challenges, enabling her to regain confidence and return to a fulfilling life.

Conclusion

Treatment for Gerstmann's Syndrome is multifaceted, requiring attention to its underlying causes, symptom management through therapies, and the potential use of supportive medications. With advances in medical technology and research, the future holds promise for more targeted treatments, offering hope to patients and their families. A multidisciplinary care team remains essential to navigating this complex condition, ensuring that each patient receives personalized and comprehensive care.

References

1. Patil VC, Kulkarni AR. Gerstmann's Syndrome: A Rare Clinical Condition with a Tetrad of Symptoms. Int J Contemp Med Surg Radiol. 2019;4(2):B173-175.

2. Toader C, Brehar FM, Radoi MP, et al. The Management of a Giant Convexity en Plaque Anaplastic Meningioma with Gerstmann Syndrome: A Case Report of Surgical Outcomes. Diagnostics (Basel). 2024;14(2566):1-12.

3. Alare K, Abioye E, Saydo B. Gerstmann Syndrome: What is the Possible Role of Deep Brain Stimulation? Neurocrit Care. 2024.

4. Yoon SH, Lee JI, Kang MJ, et al. Gerstmann Syndrome as a Disconnection Syndrome: A Single Case Diffusion Tensor Imaging Study. Brain Neurorehabil. 2023;16(1):e3.

7 Living with Gerstmann's Syndrome

Living with Gerstmann's Syndrome is a journey of adaptation and resilience. The syndrome's impact on daily life, from difficulty recognizing fingers to struggles with writing and math, can be overwhelming for patients and families alike. However, with the right strategies, tools, and support systems, individuals can navigate these challenges and lead fulfilling lives. This chapter provides practical advice and highlights the importance of therapy, community, and personalized coping techniques.

Strategies for Coping with Daily Challenges

Coping with Gerstmann's Syndrome begins with acknowledging the unique ways it affects each person. For many, the key lies in breaking tasks into manageable steps and finding creative solutions to everyday obstacles.

- **Overcoming Finger Agnosia**: Finger agnosia, or difficulty identifying one's fingers, can interfere with tasks like typing or playing an instrument. Simple strategies, such as wearing rings or color-coding fingers with nail polish, can help individuals differentiate between them. Maria, a piano teacher, relied on small stickers on her fingers during lessons to regain confidence while playing.

• **Addressing Dysgraphia**: Writing challenges can be mitigated through adaptive tools like speech-to-text software, specially designed pens, or keyboards with larger keys. Alex, a writer with Gerstmann's Syndrome, switched to dictation apps to compose articles, enabling him to continue his career without the frustration of handwriting.

• **Managing Dyscalculia**: Calculating even basic numbers can be daunting for those with Gerstmann's Syndrome. Visual aids, calculators, and apps that simplify mathematical tasks are invaluable. Lily, a student struggling with math, found success using a tactile number line and a visual calculator app designed for children.

• **Navigating Right-Left Disorientation**: To address spatial confusion, individuals can rely on mnemonics or wearable reminders, such as wristbands on their dominant hand. Techniques like consistent labeling of objects (e.g., "right" and "left" shoes) can also alleviate daily frustrations.

Each strategy emphasizes the importance of patience and persistence. Adopting a trial-and-error approach allows patients to discover what works best for their unique needs.

Tools and Resources for Managing Symptoms

Technological advancements and accessible resources play a vital role in helping individuals manage Gerstmann's Syndrome. These tools not only support day-to-day functioning but also empower patients to regain independence.

• **Assistive Technology**: Innovations in technology have revolutionized how individuals cope with the syndrome's challenges. Apps that assist with writing, such as Grammarly or speech-to-text converters, simplify communication. Math-focused programs, like Photomath or interactive calculators, are tailored to support dyscalculia.

- **Adaptive Devices**: Tools like ergonomic pens, finger guides, and color-coded keyboards enhance functionality for specific tasks. Liam, a student with developmental Gerstmann's Syndrome, used custom grips on pencils to improve his handwriting while mastering fine motor skills.

- **Educational Resources**: Online platforms and support groups provide valuable information and advice for families navigating Gerstmann's Syndrome. Parents of children with the syndrome can access forums, webinars, and learning materials that address educational challenges.

- **Visual Aids**: Charts, diagrams, and color-coded reminders are essential tools for overcoming disorientation and memory lapses. For example, maps with directional arrows help individuals struggling with right-left confusion.

These resources empower individuals to overcome limitations and approach life with renewed confidence.

Support Systems for Patients and Families

The importance of a robust support system cannot be overstated when living with Gerstmann's Syndrome. Patients thrive when surrounded by understanding and encouragement from family, friends, and professionals.

- **Family Support**: Families play a central role in fostering a positive environment. Open communication, shared problem-solving, and patience go a long way in reducing frustration. Maria's family created a structured routine that included labeled household items, making her daily activities more manageable.

- **Peer Support Groups**: Connecting with others facing similar challenges offers emotional relief and practical insights. Support groups, whether in-person or online, provide a platform for sharing experiences, exchanging tips, and building a sense of community.

- **Professional Guidance**: Psychologists, occupational therapists, and educational specialists offer tailored interventions to address specific needs. Regular therapy sessions help patients develop coping mechanisms and achieve personal goals.

- **Educational Advocacy**: For children, teachers and school counselors play a critical role in creating an inclusive learning environment. Individualized Education Programs (IEPs) and accommodations, such as extra time for tasks, are essential for academic success.

Support systems provide a safety net, reminding patients and families that they are not alone in their journey.

The Role of Therapy in Improving Quality of Life

Therapy is a cornerstone of living with Gerstmann's Syndrome, addressing both the physical and emotional aspects of the condition. A multidisciplinary approach ensures comprehensive care.

- **Occupational Therapy**: Occupational therapists focus on improving fine motor skills and adapting daily routines to the patient's abilities. Alex worked with an occupational therapist to master using assistive tools, such as adaptive keyboards and specialized calculators, to enhance his productivity.

- **Speech and Language Therapy**: For patients with writing difficulties, speech therapists provide strategies to improve communication. Techniques like using alternative communication methods or building vocabulary help individuals express themselves effectively.

- **Cognitive Behavioral Therapy (CBT)**: Emotional challenges, such as frustration and anxiety, often accompany the syndrome. CBT equips patients with techniques to manage stress, build resilience, and maintain a positive outlook.

- **Educational Therapy**: Children benefit from therapy tailored to their developmental needs, incorporating play-based learning and multisensory techniques. Lily's therapist used creative games to teach math concepts, transforming her approach to learning.

Therapy offers patients the tools to navigate their world with greater ease, fostering independence and self-confidence.

Conclusion

Living with Gerstmann's Syndrome presents unique challenges, but it also offers opportunities for growth, adaptation, and resilience. By embracing strategies for coping, leveraging tools and resources, and building strong support systems, individuals can overcome obstacles and thrive. Therapy serves as a transformative force, improving both functional abilities and emotional well-being. Together, these elements empower patients and families to face the condition with strength and optimism, creating a pathway to a fulfilling life.

8 Developmental Gerstmann's Syndrome

Developmental Gerstmann's Syndrome (DGS) represents a unique subset of learning disabilities, distinct from the acquired form typically seen in adults. While the hallmark symptoms—finger agnosia, dysgraphia, dyscalculia, and left-right disorientation—are shared, DGS arises from atypical neurodevelopment rather than acquired brain lesions. Its subtle yet pervasive effects on cognition, motor skills, and sensory integration make it a challenging condition to diagnose and manage. This chapter delves into the clinical features of DGS, its neurological underpinnings, and the importance of early intervention in fostering success for affected children.

Understanding Developmental Gerstmann's Syndrome

Unlike its acquired counterpart, DGS manifests during childhood as a developmental anomaly, often presenting as learning difficulties. It is frequently misdiagnosed as general dyslexia or other learning disorders due to overlapping symptoms. However, distinct features—such as the combination of finger agnosia with acalculia and agraphia with right-left disorientation—set DGS apart as a specific clinical entity.

Children with DGS often show no structural abnormalities on imaging, yet they exhibit functional deficits in the parietal lobe, particularly in the angular gyrus. Subtle motor and sensory impairments, including graphesthesia challenges and time disorientation, further complicate the clinical picture. For many children, these symptoms go unnoticed unless actively assessed by clinicians familiar with the condition.

Neurological Basis and Theoretical Insights

DGS offers fascinating insights into brain development and the interconnectedness of cognitive processes. The parietal lobe's role in integrating sensory input with motor planning, numerical understanding, and spatial orientation becomes evident through the unique symptom clusters observed in DGS.

- **Associations Between Symptoms**: The co-occurrence of finger agnosia with acalculia and agraphia with right-left disorientation reflects specific disruptions in neuropsychological processing. For example, difficulties in identifying fingers may hinder the development of numerical skills, as counting often relies on finger-based strategies in early childhood.

- **Dissociation of Oral and Written Language**: Many children with DGS demonstrate a striking disparity between oral communication, which remains intact, and written language, which is severely impaired. This dissociation sheds light on the brain's compartmentalization of language processing and its reliance on distinct neural circuits.

Lily, a 10-year-old with DGS, exemplified this disparity. While she excelled in verbal storytelling, her writing was illegible, and her numerical skills lagged significantly behind her peers. Her case underscored the need for tailored educational strategies that build on oral strengths while addressing written deficits.

Distinct Features of Developmental Gerstmann's Syndrome

- **Motor and Sensory Impairments**: Children with DGS often display subtle neurological signs, such as motor incoordination, impaired graphesthesia, and abnormal reflexes. These deficits suggest poor maturation of the nervous system, further complicating the development of fine motor and cognitive skills.

- **Behavioral and Emotional Challenges**: Frustration from academic struggles can lead to behavioral issues and low self-esteem. Parents and teachers frequently report emotional outbursts or withdrawal, highlighting the importance of addressing both the academic and emotional needs of these children.

Ben, an 8-year-old with DGS, struggled with tying his shoes and identifying his left from his right, leading to frequent frustration in class. His teacher, unaware of his condition, initially labeled him as inattentive. Following a diagnosis, interventions focusing on sensory integration and spatial awareness dramatically improved Ben's confidence and classroom behavior.

- **Impact of Multilingual Environments**: In cultures requiring biliteracy or triliteracy, the challenges of DGS are magnified. The additional cognitive load of learning multiple scripts and languages exacerbates difficulties with writing and spatial orientation, often delaying literacy development.

Diagnosis and Early Identification

Diagnosing DGS requires a thorough evaluation of the characteristic symptoms alongside a detailed neurological and developmental history. Many cases remain undiagnosed due to a lack of awareness among educators and clinicians. Standardized testing for fine motor skills, numerical reasoning, and spatial orientation is critical in identifying DGS early.

Maria, a mother of a 7-year-old boy with DGS, sought help after noticing her son's persistent struggles with handwriting and math. A neuropsychological assessment revealed the classic tetrad of symptoms, leading to a formal diagnosis. Early identification allowed her son to receive targeted therapies, significantly improving his academic performance.

Intervention and Treatment Strategies

The cornerstone of managing DGS lies in early and intensive intervention. Tailored therapies address the specific deficits associated with the syndrome, while adaptive strategies empower children to overcome daily challenges.

- **Occupational Therapy**: Focused on improving fine motor coordination, occupational therapy helps children develop the skills necessary for writing and other manual tasks. Exercises involving finger identification and tactile stimulation are particularly beneficial.

- **Educational Support**: Individualized Education Programs (IEPs) and classroom accommodations ensure that children with DGS receive the support they need. Tools like visual aids, interactive math programs, and assistive writing devices help mitigate academic challenges.

- **Speech and Language Therapy**: For children with significant agraphia, speech and language therapists develop alternative communication strategies, such as dictation tools or structured writing exercises.

- **Parent and Teacher Training**: Educating parents and teachers about DGS equips them to provide consistent support at home and in the classroom.

Workshops and seminars on recognizing and managing DGS foster a collaborative approach to care.

Patient Stories: The Power of Early Intervention

- **Liam's Progress**: Diagnosed at age 6, Liam initially struggled with basic math and writing. His parents enrolled him in a program combining occupational therapy with interactive learning tools. Over time, Liam gained confidence in his abilities, earning praise from his teachers and peers.

- **Emily's Breakthrough**: Emily, an 11-year-old bilingual student, faced unique challenges due to the demands of learning two languages. Intensive therapy focusing on her fine motor skills and spatial awareness helped Emily master reading and writing in both languages, proving that with the right support, children with DGS can thrive.

Future Directions in Research and Care

Ongoing research into DGS aims to uncover the neurological mechanisms underlying its unique symptom clusters. Advances in neuroimaging, such as functional MRI and diffusion tensor imaging, hold promise for identifying subtle brain abnormalities associated with DGS. Additionally, innovative therapies, including virtual reality-based cognitive training, are being explored as potential tools for enhancing spatial and numerical skills.

Advocacy efforts by families and organizations play a crucial role in driving research and raising awareness about DGS. By fostering collaboration between clinicians, educators, and researchers, these efforts ensure that children with DGS receive the care and resources they need to succeed.

Conclusion

Developmental Gerstmann's Syndrome is a complex yet fascinating condition that highlights the intricate interplay between brain development and cognitive functioning. By recognizing its distinct features and addressing the unique needs of affected children, clinicians, educators, and families can unlock their potential. Early identification, targeted interventions, and continued research pave the way for brighter futures, ensuring that children with DGS thrive both academically and personally.

References

1. Suresh PA, Sebastian S. Developmental Gerstmann's syndrome: a distinct clinical entity of learning disabilities. *Pediatr Neurol.* 2000;22(4):267-278. doi:10.1016/S0887-8994(99)00157-5.

9 Children and Education

Education plays a vital role in helping children with Gerstmann's Syndrome navigate their challenges and achieve their potential. The syndrome's characteristic difficulties with math, writing, and spatial orientation can pose significant barriers in the classroom, but with the right strategies, these barriers can be transformed into opportunities for growth. This chapter explores how to support children with Gerstmann's Syndrome in an educational setting, adapt teaching methods, and empower parents to advocate for their children effectively.

Helping Children with Gerstmann's Syndrome Succeed in School

For children with Gerstmann's Syndrome, school can be both a source of frustration and an arena for incredible growth. The challenges they face are often misunderstood or mistaken for general learning difficulties, leading to delays in receiving appropriate support. Early identification and targeted intervention are critical to fostering their success.

- **Recognizing Challenges Early**: Teachers and parents may first notice issues with fine motor skills, such as trouble holding a pencil or forming letters, as well as struggles with basic math concepts. These challenges often manifest in kindergarten or early elementary school, making early diagnosis crucial.

- **Building Confidence**: Many children with Gerstmann's Syndrome experience low self-esteem due to their difficulties in keeping up with peers. Teachers can help by celebrating small achievements, providing positive reinforcement, and creating an inclusive environment that emphasizes each child's unique strengths.

Lily, a nine-year-old with developmental Gerstmann's Syndrome, faced persistent challenges in math and handwriting, which deeply affected her confidence in school. Simple tasks like solving basic arithmetic problems or forming legible letters often left her frustrated and disheartened. Recognizing Lily's struggles, her teacher implemented a reward system that emphasized effort rather than accuracy. This shift in focus allowed Lily to celebrate small victories, such as completing an assignment or attempting a new problem. Over time, she began to feel proud of her progress and remained motivated to tackle more challenging tasks, fostering both her confidence and resilience.

Creating a nurturing environment, her classroom displayed colorful charts and tools to support her learning, with visual aids and interactive games playing a central role in helping Lily grasp concepts that once seemed out of reach.

- **Encouraging Collaboration**: Pairing children with Gerstmann's Syndrome with supportive peers fosters a sense of belonging and promotes cooperative learning. Group activities that emphasize teamwork rather than individual performance can help children feel valued.

Adapting Teaching Methods and Classroom Strategies

Teachers play a pivotal role in helping children with Gerstmann's Syndrome overcome their academic challenges. By tailoring classroom strategies to the child's needs, educators can create an environment where these children can thrive.

- **Math Instruction**: Dyscalculia, a core feature of Gerstmann's Syndrome, requires creative teaching approaches. Visual aids, tactile tools like counting blocks, and step-by-step instruction are invaluable. Teachers can use apps and software designed to simplify math concepts, allowing students to grasp abstract ideas through interactive, engaging methods.

Ben, a ten-year-old with Gerstmann's Syndrome, struggled with basic arithmetic. His teacher introduced manipulatives like beads and number lines, which helped him visualize problems and build confidence in his math skills.

- **Handwriting Support**: For children with dysgraphia, writing tasks can be daunting. Teachers can provide assistive tools such as pencil grips, specialized paper with bold lines, or technology like tablets with handwriting apps. Encouraging alternative methods of expression, such as typing or dictation, ensures children can focus on content rather than form.

- **Spatial Orientation**: Left-right disorientation and difficulties with spatial relationships can make navigation and map reading challenging. Teachers can use visual cues, such as labeled classroom objects or directional arrows, to reduce confusion. Incorporating consistent routines helps children feel grounded and oriented.

- **Differentiated Instruction**: Adapting lesson plans to the child's learning pace and style is critical. Breaking tasks into smaller, manageable steps allows children to process information without feeling overwhelmed. Providing extra time for assignments and tests accommodates their need for additional processing time.

- **Interactive Learning**: Engaging children in hands-on activities, such as building models or exploring geometry through physical objects, can enhance understanding. These approaches are particularly helpful for children who struggle with abstract concepts.

Educational Resources and Advocacy for Parents

Parents of children with Gerstmann's Syndrome play a crucial role in ensuring their children receive the support they need. Accessing resources, advocating for accommodations, and fostering communication between home and school are essential components of this process.

- **Individualized Education Programs (IEPs)**: IEPs are tailored plans that outline specific goals and accommodations for children with special needs. Parents should collaborate with teachers, school psychologists, and therapists to develop an IEP that addresses their child's unique challenges. Accommodations might include extra time for tests, reduced writing demands, or access to technology for assignments.

- **Parent-Teacher Communication**: Regular communication between parents and teachers helps ensure consistency in addressing the child's needs. Sharing updates on progress, challenges, and strategies allows for a unified approach to support.

- **Workshops and Seminars**: Parents can benefit from attending workshops that provide insights into Gerstmann's Syndrome and effective advocacy techniques. These events often connect families with specialists and other parents facing similar challenges, creating a supportive community.

- **At-Home Support**: Parents can reinforce classroom strategies at home by incorporating learning activities into daily routines. Simple tasks like cooking can become opportunities to practice math, while board games can enhance spatial awareness and collaboration.

- **Online Resources and Communities**: Websites, forums, and social media groups dedicated to learning disabilities and Gerstmann's Syndrome offer valuable advice and emotional support. Parents can access toolkits, find recommended apps, and connect with experts in the field.

When Liam's parents joined an online forum for families dealing with Gerstmann's Syndrome, they discovered new strategies for managing his dyscalculia. The connections they made provided not only practical tips but also reassurance that they were not alone in their journey.

Advocating for Change

Advocating for children with Gerstmann's Syndrome extends beyond the classroom. Parents and educators can work together to raise awareness and push for systemic changes that benefit all students with learning challenges.

- **Training for Educators**: Many teachers lack training in recognizing and addressing the specific needs of children with Gerstmann's Syndrome. Advocacy efforts should focus on professional development programs that equip educators with the knowledge and tools to support these students.

- **Policy Changes**: Parents can join forces with advocacy groups to influence education policies that promote inclusivity and accessibility. Efforts might include lobbying for increased funding for special education or the inclusion of Gerstmann's Syndrome in diagnostic and educational guidelines.

- **Awareness Campaigns**: Increasing awareness about Gerstmann's Syndrome through community events, social media, and school presentations helps reduce stigma and foster understanding. By sharing stories and successes, families can inspire empathy and support.

Conclusion

Education is a powerful tool for children with Gerstmann's Syndrome, offering them the chance to overcome challenges and reach their potential. With the right teaching methods, classroom adaptations, and parental advocacy, these children can thrive academically and personally. By fostering collaboration between educators, families, and the community, we create an environment where every child can succeed, regardless of the obstacles they face. Through resilience, creativity, and determination, children with Gerstmann's Syndrome can build a bright and promising future.

10 Navigating Relationships and Communication

Relationships form the foundation of emotional resilience for individuals living with Gerstmann's Syndrome. The condition's challenges, such as difficulties with writing, math, and spatial awareness, can strain communication and understanding between patients and their loved ones. However, with open dialogue, empathy, and the support of communities, these relationships can become a source of strength and encouragement. This chapter explores strategies for explaining Gerstmann's Syndrome to family and friends, strengthening patient-family bonds, and finding support groups that foster connection and understanding.

Explaining the Condition to Family and Friends

One of the first steps in navigating relationships is helping others understand what Gerstmann's Syndrome entails. Many people, even within the patient's closest circle, may not be familiar with the condition, leading to confusion or misconceptions about its impact. Clear, honest communication is key to fostering empathy and support.

- **Breaking Down the Symptoms**:

Explaining the four hallmark symptoms—finger agnosia, dysgraphia, dyscalculia, and left-right disorientation—provides a concrete foundation for understanding. Using relatable examples can make the condition more accessible. For instance, describing how dyscalculia makes simple tasks like counting change challenging helps illustrate the daily struggles a patient may face.

- **Using Analogies**: Analogies can simplify complex concepts. For example, explaining dysgraphia as the brain knowing what it wants to write but struggling to communicate that message to the hand can help loved ones grasp the frustration patients feel.

- **Sharing Patient Stories**: Personal experiences are powerful tools for fostering understanding. When Alex, a father of two, was diagnosed with Gerstmann's Syndrome after a stroke, he shared his challenges with writing and distinguishing his left from his right. By openly discussing his difficulties, he helped his family see the condition not as a limitation but as a new way of navigating life.

- **Providing Educational Materials**: Sharing articles, videos, or books about Gerstmann's Syndrome can help family and friends learn at their own pace. This approach also alleviates the burden on the patient to explain every detail.

Strengthening Patient-Family Relationships

Living with Gerstmann's Syndrome can test even the strongest relationships. Families often need to adapt their routines and expectations, which can lead to frustration or feelings of helplessness. However, with effort and understanding, these challenges can bring families closer together.

- **Practicing Patience and Empathy**: Patients may take longer to complete tasks or need extra help with daily activities. Patience is essential in supporting their journey. For example, Maria, whose husband struggles with dysgraphia, often helps him write letters and fill out forms. She views these moments as opportunities to bond rather than as burdens.

- **Celebrating Small Victories**: Acknowledging progress, no matter how minor, boosts morale for both the patient and their family. When Liam, a young boy with Gerstmann's Syndrome, learned to tie his shoes independently after months of practice, his family threw a small celebration to honor his achievement.

- **Creating a Supportive Environment**: Families can take proactive steps to adapt their homes in ways that make life significantly easier for individuals living with Gerstmann's Syndrome. By creating an environment tailored to the patient's specific needs, they can help reduce daily stress and frustration, fostering a greater sense of comfort and independence. Simple yet effective changes, such as labeling household items with clear text or images and incorporating visual cues like arrows or color codes, can alleviate confusion and streamline routines. For example, assigning specific colors to different household tasks or tools can help patients identify and use them more easily without the added pressure of figuring things out on their own.

Maggie, a devoted mother of three, took this approach to heart by introducing a comprehensive color-coded system in her home. Each family member was assigned a color, which Maggie used to label items such as towels, toothbrushes, and even kitchen drawers. Additionally, she implemented visual reminders on walls and doors to guide her daughter through daily tasks, such as dressing or organizing school supplies. These thoughtful adaptations not only simplified her daughter's routines but also instilled a newfound sense of independence and confidence, enabling her to take charge of her responsibilities with less reliance on constant assistance.

- **Encouraging Open Communication**: Regularly checking in with the patient about their feelings and needs helps prevent misunderstandings. Creating a safe space for open dialogue allows patients to express their frustrations and seek support without fear of judgment.

Finding and Participating in Support Groups

Support groups offer invaluable opportunities for patients and families to connect with others who share similar experiences. These communities provide a space for sharing advice, gaining insights, and building friendships that can last a lifetime.

- **Benefits of Support Groups**: For patients, these groups provide validation and reduce feelings of isolation. Hearing others share their struggles and triumphs fosters a sense of belonging. For families, support groups offer practical advice and emotional reassurance.

- **Types of Support Groups**: Support groups can take many forms, from in-person meetings to online forums and social media communities. Each offers unique benefits, allowing participants to choose the format that best suits their needs.

- **Finding the Right Group**: Patients and families should seek out groups tailored to their experiences. For example, parents of children with Gerstmann's Syndrome may benefit from forums focused on educational strategies and parenting tips, while adults with the condition might prefer groups that address workplace accommodations and daily living.

- **Building Community Connections**: Beyond formal support groups, patients and families can find support in their local communities. Joining clubs, participating in volunteer activities, or attending workshops can help them build meaningful relationships and expand their network.

Lily's mother found immense comfort in an online community for parents of children with learning disabilities. Through the group, she discovered new strategies for managing Lily's dyscalculia and connected with other parents who understood her journey. These relationships became a lifeline during challenging times.

Strength Through Shared Experiences

Patient stories illustrate the power of relationships and community in navigating Gerstmann's Syndrome. Alex's journey of opening up to his family allowed them to work together to address his challenges. Liam's achievements, celebrated by his supportive family, showed the value of encouragement and patience. Lily's mother's connection to a wider network of parents demonstrated how shared experiences can foster hope and resilience.

Conclusion

Navigating relationships and communication with Gerstmann's Syndrome requires effort, empathy, and a willingness to adapt. By fostering understanding among family and friends, strengthening bonds through patience and support, and seeking connections within the community, patients and their loved ones can create a network of care and encouragement. These relationships not only help manage the challenges of the condition but also serve as a source of strength, empowering patients to lead fulfilling lives.

11 Advances in Research

In recent years, understanding the intricacies of Gerstmann's Syndrome has evolved significantly. Once considered an obscure neurological condition with four hallmark symptoms—finger agnosia, dysgraphia, dyscalculia, and left-right disorientation—it is now recognized as a window into the complexities of brain functionality. With advancements in neuroimaging and neuropsychological testing, researchers have identified that the angular gyrus in the parietal lobe is central to the manifestation of this syndrome. These breakthroughs have refined diagnostic criteria and enabled more precise differentiation from other neurological disorders.

One patient, Thomas, a retired architect, highlighted the importance of early identification. After a minor stroke, he noticed difficulties writing and distinguishing his left from his right. Initially dismissed as stress, his symptoms were later identified as part of Gerstmann's Syndrome through advanced imaging and neurocognitive assessments. His case underscores how enhanced diagnostic tools can change lives, allowing for targeted interventions that improve daily functioning.

Emerging Treatments and Therapies

Treatment for Gerstmann's Syndrome has transitioned from symptom management to exploring therapies targeting the underlying neural disruptions. Cognitive rehabilitation, occupational therapy, and tailored educational strategies have proven effective in enhancing the quality of life for patients. Emerging research is focusing on neuroplasticity, aiming to retrain the brain to compensate for deficits caused by damage to the angular gyrus.

Consider Emily, a 12-year-old struggling with dyscalculia and dysgraphia. Her family enrolled her in a research trial utilizing virtual reality (VR) for cognitive training. The program presented immersive tasks requiring spatial navigation and problem-solving, which strengthened her neural pathways. Emily's remarkable progress—writing short essays and solving basic math problems—offers hope for innovative therapies redefining patient care.

The Role of Patient Advocacy in Research

Patient advocacy groups have emerged as powerful catalysts for advancing research into rare conditions like Gerstmann's Syndrome. By uniting patients, families, and clinicians, these groups amplify voices that often go unheard in the broader medical community. Advocacy organizations are instrumental in securing funding, promoting awareness, and driving clinical trials.

One poignant example is the Johnson family, who founded an advocacy group after their son was diagnosed with developmental Gerstmann's Syndrome. Their grassroots efforts have raised significant funds for research and connected hundreds of families with resources. Their work illustrates how collective action can spark progress, bringing attention to conditions that might otherwise remain in the shadows.

Current Clinical Trials and How to Participate

Clinical trials are the cornerstone of medical advancements, offering a glimpse into the future of treatment and care for Gerstmann's Syndrome. Trials investigating non-invasive brain stimulation, pharmacological interventions, and AI-driven diagnostic tools are ongoing, with preliminary results showing promise.

John, a 50-year-old accountant, became involved in a clinical trial exploring transcranial magnetic stimulation (TMS) for cognitive enhancement. Over 12 weeks, he reported significant improvements in spatial awareness and handwriting, allowing him to return to work part-time. His participation not only benefited him personally but contributed valuable data for refining this experimental therapy.

For families seeking to join trials, the process often begins with consulting specialists or exploring online registries. While participation requires commitment, many patients and families find the opportunity to contribute to scientific progress profoundly rewarding.

Conclusion

The future of Gerstmann's Syndrome research is bright, driven by advances in neuroscience, innovative therapies, and the tireless efforts of advocacy groups. By understanding the condition's neural underpinnings, exploring groundbreaking treatments, and fostering community engagement, researchers and patients are paving the way toward improved care and, ultimately, hope for those affected. The journey ahead holds promise, as each discovery brings us closer to a world where Gerstmann's Syndrome is not only understood but effectively managed.

References

1. Harding E, Sullivan MP, Camic PM, et al. Exploring experiential differences in everyday activities: A focused ethnographic study in the homes of people living

with memory-led Alzheimer's disease and posterior cortical atrophy. *Journal of Aging Studies*. 2024;69:101226.

2. Montembeault M, Migliaccio R. Atypical forms of Alzheimer's disease: patients not to forget. *Current Opinion in Neurology*. 2023;36(4):245-252.

3. Yerstein O, Parand L, Liang LJ, et al. Benson's Disease or Posterior Cortical Atrophy, revisited. *Journal of Alzheimer's Disease*. 2021;82(2):493-502.

4. Trapp NT, Martyna MR, Siddiqi SH, et al. The Neuropsychiatric Approach to the Assessment of Patients in Neurology. *Semin Neurol*. 2022;42(2):88-106.

5. Jang AI, Bernstock JD, Segar DJ, et al. Case Report: Frontoparietal Metastasis from a Primary Fallopian Tube Carcinoma. *Frontiers in Surgery*. 2021;8:594570.

12 Support and Resources

Navigating life with Gerstmann's Syndrome can feel overwhelming, but a wealth of resources exists to help patients and their families. These resources—ranging from organizations and support groups to educational websites and tips for finding specialists—provide critical support, guidance, and a sense of community. By leveraging these tools, patients and families can better understand the condition, access expert care, and connect with others facing similar challenges. This chapter highlights key resources and shares patient stories that illustrate their transformative impact.

Organizations and Support Groups

Organizations and support groups are lifelines for patients and families living with Gerstmann's Syndrome. These communities foster connection, provide reliable information, and advocate for greater awareness and research.

- **National and International Organizations**: Foundations such as the Neurological Disorders Alliance and Learning Disabilities Association offer resources tailored to specific symptoms of Gerstmann's Syndrome, such as dysgraphia or dyscalculia.

These organizations often host webinars, publish educational materials, and connect families with local services.

- **Local Support Groups**: Community-based support groups provide opportunities for in-person connection, where families can share experiences and strategies. These groups also facilitate mentorship, pairing newly diagnosed individuals with those who have successfully navigated similar challenges.

- **Online Communities**: Virtual support groups on platforms like Facebook or specialized forums offer flexibility for families who may not have access to local resources. These spaces allow participants to share tips, celebrate milestones, and provide emotional support around the clock.

For Maggie, a mother of three, joining an online group for parents of children with learning disabilities was a turning point. Through the group, she discovered new strategies for helping her son overcome dyscalculia and found comfort in hearing from other parents who truly understood her journey. The friendships she built through the group became a source of strength during tough times.

Educational Websites and Online Tools

The internet is a treasure trove of information for families navigating Gerstmann's Syndrome. From comprehensive educational websites to innovative apps, these resources empower families with knowledge and tools to manage daily challenges.

- **Condition-Specific Websites**: Websites dedicated to neurological and learning disorders, such as MedlinePlus and the National Institute of Neurological Disorders and Stroke, provide clear, accessible information about Gerstmann's Syndrome. These sites cover topics ranging from symptoms and diagnosis to emerging treatments and research.

- **Interactive Learning Apps**: Apps like Dysgraphia Hero and Photomath offer tailored exercises to support children struggling with handwriting and math. These tools use gamification to make learning engaging and effective, transforming previously daunting tasks into manageable and enjoyable activities.

- **Parent and Educator Portals**: Websites like Understood.org provide resources for parents and educators, including guides on advocating for Individualized Education Programs (IEPs), classroom accommodations, and tips for supporting children at home.

Ben, a ten-year-old with Gerstmann's Syndrome, thrived after his family discovered an app that turned math problems into interactive puzzles. By gamifying math, the app helped Ben build confidence and improve his skills while having fun. His mother noted that the app also sparked discussions at school, where teachers began incorporating similar tools into the classroom.

Tips for Finding Specialists and Care Providers

Access to knowledgeable specialists and care providers is essential for managing Gerstmann's Syndrome effectively. However, finding the right professionals can be daunting, especially for families unfamiliar with the healthcare system. The following tips can simplify the process:

1. **Start with Referrals**: Primary care physicians or pediatricians are excellent starting points for referrals to neurologists, neuropsychologists, or therapists with experience in conditions like Gerstmann's Syndrome.

2. **Search Specialized Directories**: Professional organizations, such as the American Academy of Neurology or the American Occupational Therapy Association, maintain directories of certified providers. Searching these databases by location and specialty can help narrow down options.

3. **Leverage Local Resources**: Hospitals, clinics, and community health centers often have patient navigators or social workers who can guide families to the appropriate specialists.

4. **Connect with Advocacy Groups**: Advocacy organizations often maintain lists of trusted care providers. Additionally, connecting with other families in support groups can yield valuable recommendations.

5. **Ask Questions**: When meeting potential specialists, don't hesitate to ask about their experience with Gerstmann's Syndrome or similar conditions. Understanding their approach to treatment and their familiarity with the syndrome ensures alignment with the patient's needs.

Emily, a teenager diagnosed with Gerstmann's Syndrome, found life-changing support through a neuropsychologist her family discovered on an advocacy group's website. The psychologist's personalized approach helped Emily develop coping strategies, boosting her academic performance and confidence.

Patient Stories: The Power of Connection

Patient stories illuminate how accessing the right resources can transform lives.

- **Maria's Journey**: Maria, a retired teacher, initially felt isolated after her diagnosis. A friend encouraged her to join a local support group, where she met others facing similar challenges. The group introduced her to assistive tools that simplified daily tasks and inspired her to advocate for others with Gerstmann's Syndrome.

- **Liam's Success**: Liam, a young boy struggling with dysgraphia and dyscalculia, benefited from a combination of educational apps and occupational therapy. His parents discovered these resources through a webinar hosted by a national organization. Liam's progress, celebrated by his family and teachers, demonstrates the importance of early intervention and consistent support.

- **Alex's Advocacy**: Alex, a stroke survivor, used his experience with Gerstmann's Syndrome to raise awareness about the condition. By sharing his story through an online blog, he connected with readers worldwide, fostering understanding and empathy while offering practical advice for navigating life with the syndrome.

Building a Network of Support

The key to thriving with Gerstmann's Syndrome lies in building a strong network of support. This network encompasses not only family and friends but also healthcare providers, educators, and advocacy communities. By tapping into the wealth of resources available, patients and their families can find guidance, encouragement, and a sense of belonging.

For patients like Lily, a young girl whose challenges once felt insurmountable, these connections have made all the difference. With the help of supportive teachers, an understanding family, and tools tailored to her needs, Lily has grown into a confident student, proving that with the right resources, anything is possible.

Conclusion

Living with Gerstmann's Syndrome can be challenging, but no one has to face it alone. Organizations, online tools, and dedicated specialists provide invaluable support, helping patients and families navigate the complexities of the condition. By sharing knowledge, fostering connections, and advocating for change, these resources create a foundation of hope and empowerment. Together, they ensure that patients with Gerstmann's Syndrome—and their families—can thrive.

13 The History of GS

The history of Gerstmann's Syndrome is a tale that reflects the evolving nature of neuropsychology. First described by Josef Gerstmann in 1924, this rare condition, characterized by the now-famous tetrad of symptoms—finger agnosia, agraphia, dyscalculia, and left-right disorientation—has sparked decades of debate and intrigue. Gerstmann, an Austrian neurologist, observed these symptoms in patients with lesions in the dominant parietal lobe and hypothesized that they stemmed from damage to a common functional denominator within this brain region. While his ideas were revolutionary for their time, they were also met with skepticism and controversy, which persist to some extent today.

The Early Years: Gerstmann's Observations

Josef Gerstmann first presented his findings in the early 1920s while working as a young assistant in Vienna. His meticulous case studies described patients who exhibited specific cognitive deficits following parietal lobe damage. At the heart of his theory was the idea that the angular gyrus played a crucial role in integrating sensory input with higher-order functions, such as recognizing one's fingers, performing arithmetic, and orienting spatially. This conceptualization of the syndrome was groundbreaking, particularly as it linked seemingly disparate symptoms to a single neurological origin.

Initially, Gerstmann's findings were met with quiet curiosity but little fanfare. His work gained more attention when he expanded his observations and proposed the idea of a distinct "syndromal entity." However, the scientific community of the time was cautious in embracing such a novel concept, particularly as neurological research was still in its infancy compared to today's standards.

The Mid-20th Century: A Turning Point

The 1950s marked a pivotal period for Gerstmann's Syndrome as neurologists and psychologists began to explore its implications more deeply. Notably, MacDonald Critchley, one of the most influential neurologists of the time, initially supported Gerstmann's theories in his seminal 1953 monograph on the parietal lobes. Critchley's endorsement brought a degree of legitimacy to the syndrome, and it began appearing more frequently in textbooks as an example of parietal lobe pathology.

However, the tide turned dramatically in 1966 when Critchley delivered his Gowers lecture. Influenced by the arguments of Arthur L. Benton, an American neuropsychologist who vehemently challenged the existence of Gerstmann's Syndrome as a coherent entity, Critchley publicly recanted much of his earlier support. Benton's critiques were rooted in the lack of consistent evidence for Gerstmann's proposed "common denominator" and the variability of symptom presentations in patients. Critchley's Gowers lecture effectively cast doubt on the syndrome's validity, leading to a decline in its acceptance among neurologists.

The Debate Intensifies

The skepticism surrounding Gerstmann's Syndrome did not deter all researchers. During the 1980s and early 1990s, fresh evidence emerged that reignited interest in the condition. Studies identifying "pure cases" of Gerstmann's Syndrome, where all four symptoms occurred without additional neurological impairments, provided compelling support for its status as a genuine syndrome. Benton himself revisited his earlier critiques and acknowledged the legitimacy of the syndrome in 1992, though he maintained that the search for a singular neurological basis for the tetrad was likely misguided.

Meanwhile, research into the angular gyrus and parietal lobe continued to evolve. Advances in neuroimaging provided new insights into the functional and structural organization of the brain, challenging and refining earlier theories. Some studies suggested that Gerstmann's Syndrome might arise not from a single lesion but from disruptions to interconnected fiber tracts within the parietal white matter.

Modern Perspectives: A Case Study in Neuropsychology

Today, Gerstmann's Syndrome occupies a unique place in neuropsychology. While no longer as contentious as it was in the mid-20th century, the syndrome remains a subject of fascination and ongoing research. It is often viewed as a case study in the dialectic evolution of scientific concepts—an example of how new evidence and perspectives can reshape our understanding of the brain.

Modern researchers continue to delve deeper into the neurological underpinnings of Gerstmann's Syndrome, with some proposing that the tetrad of symptoms—finger agnosia, agraphia, dyscalculia, and left-right disorientation—may be better understood as a disconnection syndrome rather than the result of damage to a singular cortical area. This evolving perspective shifts the focus from isolated brain regions to the intricate web of neural networks that integrate sensory, motor, and cognitive processes. Advanced imaging techniques, such as functional MRI and diffusion tensor imaging, have provided compelling evidence to support this hypothesis. These technologies reveal the interconnected pathways within the parietal lobe, highlighting how disruptions to these connections could manifest as the hallmark symptoms of Gerstmann's Syndrome. Furthermore, this approach underscores the importance of viewing the brain as a dynamic system where even minor lesions can have widespread effects, depending on the networks they disrupt. By embracing this more holistic understanding, researchers are not only refining the diagnosis of Gerstmann's Syndrome but also opening new avenues for targeted treatments that address the condition's root causes at a network level rather than focusing solely on localized damage. This paradigm shift reflects a broader trend in neuroscience, emphasizing connectivity and integration as fundamental principles of brain function.

The history of Gerstmann's Syndrome also underscores the importance of interdisciplinary collaboration in advancing medical knowledge. From Josef Gerstmann's pioneering case studies to the critiques of Benton and Critchley, and the contributions of contemporary neuroscientists, the syndrome has served as a focal point for discussions about brain function, symptom classification, and the nature of syndromal constructs.

Conclusion

The journey of Gerstmann's Syndrome from its initial description in 1924 to its current status as a recognized but still enigmatic condition reflects the broader evolution of neuropsychology. Josef Gerstmann's insights laid the groundwork for decades of research, debate, and discovery, highlighting the interconnectedness of sensory, motor, and cognitive processes within the brain. While many questions remain unanswered, the syndrome continues to inspire scientific inquiry and serves as a reminder of the complexities and mysteries of the human mind.

References

1. Rusconi E, Pinel P, Dehaene S, Kleinschmidt A. The enigma of Gerstmann's syndrome revisited: a telling tale of the vicissitudes of neuropsychology. *Brain*. 2010;133(2):320-332. doi:10.1093/brain/awp281.

2. Critchley M. The parietal lobes. London: Edward Arnold; 1953.

3. Benton AL, Myers R. Derangements of body scheme. *Neurology*. 1956;6(5):483-491.

4. Strub RL, Geschwind N. Gerstmann syndrome without aphasia. *Neurology*. 1983;33(6):672-682.

5. Morris HH, Lüders H, Lesser RP, Dinner DS, Klem G, Hahn JF. Gerstmann syndrome: disconnection or dysfunction of the parietal lobe? *Neurology*. 1984;34(7):936-941.

14 Patient Stories

While medical definitions and scientific theories help explain the complexities of Gerstmann's Syndrome, it is through the stories of those who live with the condition that its true impact becomes clear. Each individual's experience is unique, shaped by their personal circumstances, challenges, and resilience. These stories provide a window into the diverse ways Gerstmann's Syndrome manifests and how people adapt, thrive, and inspire.

1. Emily's Journey: Navigating Childhood Challenges

Emily was six years old when her teacher first noticed something unusual. She struggled with basic math tasks, had difficulty distinguishing her left hand from her right, and often became frustrated during writing exercises. Her parents initially chalked it up to normal developmental delays, but as Emily fell further behind her peers, they sought answers.

After numerous assessments, Emily was diagnosed with Developmental Gerstmann's Syndrome. At first, her parents felt overwhelmed, unsure of how to help her. A breakthrough came when an occupational therapist introduced Emily to hands-on learning tools like manipulatives for math and bold-lined paper for writing. Her teacher created a supportive classroom environment with visual aids and a buddy system for navigating tasks requiring spatial awareness.

Today, at 10 years old, Emily has blossomed into a confident, determined student. While she still faces challenges, her parents credit early intervention and a supportive school community for her progress. "Emily taught us to focus on what she can do, not what she can't," her mother says. "She's a fighter."

2. Alex's Story: Adapting to Life After a Stroke

Alex, a retired engineer, had always prided himself on his analytical mind. After a stroke at the age of 67, he found himself struggling with tasks that once came easily. Writing grocery lists became a chore, simple calculations baffled him, and he frequently mixed up directions. At first, his family assumed these difficulties were part of general cognitive decline. It wasn't until a neurologist conducted specialized tests that Alex received a diagnosis: Gerstmann's Syndrome.

The news was both a relief and a challenge. "At least we knew what we were dealing with," Alex recalls, "but it was hard to accept that these symptoms might not improve." With the help of a multidisciplinary care team, Alex learned to adapt. He began using apps to organize his tasks and relied on voice-to-text technology for writing. His family also played a crucial role, creating a home environment with clear labels and visual cues.

While Alex still mourns the loss of some abilities, he's found a new sense of purpose. He volunteers at a local stroke support group, sharing his journey and offering encouragement to others. "You can't change the past," he says, "but you can change how you move forward."

3. Maya's Experience: Balancing Motherhood and Diagnosis

For Maya, a 35-year-old mother of two, the signs of Gerstmann's Syndrome were subtle but persistent. She often confused left and right while giving directions, struggled with her children's math homework, and felt clumsy when attempting tasks that required fine motor skills. Her symptoms became more pronounced after a minor head injury in her late twenties, prompting her to seek medical advice.

The diagnosis of Gerstmann's Syndrome brought clarity but also a wave of emotions. "I felt like I'd been living with this invisible barrier my whole life, and suddenly it had a name," Maya explains. Determined not to let the condition define her, she sought out therapy and connected with online support groups. These communities became invaluable, offering tips, emotional support, and a sense of belonging.

Maya has since developed creative strategies to navigate her challenges. She uses color-coded reminders for organizing her home, relies on smartphone apps for navigation, and embraces mindfulness practices to manage stress. "It's not about perfection," she says. "It's about finding what works for you."

4. Ben's Struggles and Triumphs in the Classroom

Ben, a 12-year-old with Developmental Gerstmann's Syndrome, was often labeled as "lazy" or "unmotivated" in school before his diagnosis. He had trouble holding a pencil, his handwriting was nearly illegible, and math lessons left him in tears. His parents knew something was wrong but faced pushback from teachers who believed he just needed to try harder.

A neuropsychological evaluation finally revealed the truth. Armed with this new understanding, Ben's parents advocated for an Individualized Education Program (IEP) that included accommodations such as extra time on tests, access to typing tools, and one-on-one support for math. His school also implemented peer-assisted learning strategies, pairing Ben with a classmate for group projects.

The results were transformative. Ben began to regain his confidence and even developed a love for storytelling through typed assignments. "The diagnosis changed everything," his mother says. "It wasn't about lowering expectations; it was about giving Ben the tools to succeed."

5. Maria's Advocacy Journey

Maria, a 42-year-old nurse, noticed subtle issues with her motor skills and spatial orientation during her training years but dismissed them as quirks. It wasn't until she began experiencing significant difficulties after a car accident that she sought medical help. A diagnosis of Gerstmann's Syndrome explained years of challenges but also came with new struggles as she adapted to life with more pronounced symptoms.

Maria's experience as a nurse fueled her determination to advocate for others with rare neurological conditions. She joined a local advocacy group and later co-founded an online community for individuals with Gerstmann's Syndrome. Through webinars, social media campaigns, and in-person events, Maria works tirelessly to raise awareness and connect patients with resources.

"I want people to know they're not alone," Maria says. "Living with this condition can be isolating, but there's a community out there ready to support you."

6. Thomas: Rediscovering Purpose in Retirement

Thomas, a retired teacher, was diagnosed with Gerstmann's Syndrome in his late sixties after a series of symptoms began interfering with his daily life. Writing letters to his grandchildren became difficult, balancing his checkbook felt impossible, and he frequently got lost on familiar walking routes. For someone who had spent decades in a classroom, the loss of these skills was devastating.

With the support of his wife and a dedicated therapist, Thomas began to rebuild his confidence. He started using dictation software for writing and simplified his financial tasks by using budgeting apps. He also found solace in art, rediscovering his passion for painting as a form of self-expression.

Now, Thomas volunteers at a local senior center, teaching art classes and sharing his story with others. "I may have lost some skills," he says, "but I've gained a new way to connect with people and find joy."

Conclusion

These patient stories highlight the diversity of experiences within the Gerstmann's Syndrome community. While the condition presents unique challenges, it also reveals the incredible resilience and adaptability of those who live with it. From childhood struggles to late-life adjustments, these journeys demonstrate the power of understanding, support, and perseverance in overcoming obstacles and finding new ways to thrive.

15 Frequently Asked Questions

1. What are the main symptoms of Gerstmann's Syndrome?

The core symptoms of Gerstmann's Syndrome are finger agnosia (difficulty identifying one's fingers), dysgraphia (difficulty writing), dyscalculia (difficulty with math), and left-right disorientation. These symptoms may occur together or in varying combinations, depending on the severity and underlying cause. Additionally, some individuals may experience associated difficulties such as spatial awareness deficits or constructional apraxia.

For example, Maria, a teacher diagnosed with the syndrome, initially noticed difficulty in distinguishing her left from her right hand during daily tasks. This disorientation, combined with challenges in writing legibly, led to her eventual diagnosis. Understanding these symptoms helps individuals recognize potential signs and seek appropriate medical advice.

2. Can Gerstmann's Syndrome occur in children?

Yes, Gerstmann's Syndrome can present in children, often as a developmental condition rather than an acquired one. In such cases, it is commonly associated with learning disabilities. These children may face challenges with writing, understanding math, and navigating spatial relationships in school settings.

Liam, an 8-year-old, struggled with math and handwriting, which impacted his academic confidence. His parents initially thought he had general learning difficulties, but further evaluations revealed developmental Gerstmann's Syndrome. Early intervention, including occupational and educational therapies, helped Liam build coping skills and achieve academic milestones.

3. How is Gerstmann's Syndrome diagnosed?

Diagnosing Gerstmann's Syndrome involves a combination of clinical assessments, neuropsychological testing, and imaging studies like MRI or CT scans. Physicians typically evaluate the presence of the four hallmark symptoms through tasks that test finger recognition, writing ability, numerical understanding, and spatial orientation. Imaging may be used to identify any underlying brain damage, such as lesions in the angular gyrus of the parietal lobe.

For example, Alex, a stroke survivor, underwent extensive neuropsychological testing to evaluate his difficulties with writing and math. An MRI later confirmed damage to his left angular gyrus, leading to an accurate diagnosis.

4. What causes Gerstmann's Syndrome?

Gerstmann's Syndrome can be caused by various factors, including brain injuries (e.g., stroke or trauma), tumors, or neurodegenerative diseases that affect the angular gyrus. In children, it often has developmental origins, possibly linked to atypical brain development. Rare genetic conditions, such as Gerstmann-Sträussler-Scheinker Syndrome, may also produce similar symptoms.

Thomas, a retired architect, developed the syndrome after a mild stroke that impacted the left side of his brain. Understanding the underlying cause was crucial in planning his treatment and rehabilitation.

5. Is Gerstmann's Syndrome curable?

While there is no definitive cure for Gerstmann's Syndrome, many patients can improve their quality of life through targeted therapies and coping strategies. Occupational therapy, cognitive rehabilitation, and assistive tools can help manage symptoms effectively. Early intervention often yields the best outcomes, especially in children with developmental forms of the syndrome.

Emily, a 10-year-old diagnosed with developmental Gerstmann's Syndrome, showed significant progress in math and handwriting through therapy and the use of educational apps. While her symptoms persist, she has developed strategies to navigate daily challenges confidently.

6. How does Gerstmann's Syndrome affect daily life?

Gerstmann's Syndrome can impact various aspects of daily life, from performing simple tasks like tying shoes to more complex activities such as writing checks or following directions. Left-right disorientation can make navigation challenging, while dyscalculia complicates financial management.

Maggie, a retired librarian, found it difficult to follow recipes due to her trouble with numerical measurements. After adapting her kitchen with visual aids and color-coded tools, she regained independence in cooking, demonstrating how small adjustments can significantly improve daily living.

7. What treatments are available for Gerstmann's Syndrome?

Treatment focuses on managing symptoms and addressing underlying causes. Therapies such as occupational therapy, speech therapy, and cognitive rehabilitation are commonly used to help patients build skills and adapt to their challenges. Assistive tools, like ergonomic writing devices or math-oriented apps, can also provide support. In cases caused by brain injuries, addressing the primary condition—such as reducing inflammation or repairing lesions—is a critical first step.

John, a 45-year-old mechanic, worked with an occupational therapist to relearn spatial tasks after his diagnosis. Using adaptive tools and consistent practice, he was able to return to work part-time.

8. Are there support groups for individuals with Gerstmann's Syndrome?

Yes, there are support groups specifically for individuals with learning disabilities and rare neurological conditions, including Gerstmann's Syndrome. These groups provide a platform for patients and families to share experiences, offer emotional support, and exchange practical advice. Both in-person and online communities are available, offering flexibility for participants.

Maria, a mother of a child with the syndrome, joined an online group where she connected with other parents facing similar challenges. The group provided her with invaluable insights into educational strategies and fostered a sense of community.

9. How does Gerstmann's Syndrome impact education?

In children, Gerstmann's Syndrome can lead to academic struggles, particularly in subjects like math and writing. Dysgraphia may make it difficult to complete written assignments, while dyscalculia affects numerical understanding. Left-right disorientation can also interfere with navigation and spatial tasks in the classroom. Individualized Education Programs (IEPs) and tailored accommodations are crucial to supporting these students.

Ben, a 12-year-old, faced significant hurdles in school due to his difficulties with writing and math. With the help of a dedicated teacher and an IEP, he gained access to assistive tools and extra time on tests, allowing him to thrive academically.

10. Can adults develop Gerstmann's Syndrome?

Yes, Gerstmann's Syndrome can develop in adults, typically as a result of neurological events like strokes, traumatic brain injuries, or tumors. In these cases, symptoms may emerge suddenly and require immediate medical attention to prevent further complications. Rehabilitation and therapy can help adults adapt to the condition and regain independence.

Thomas, a 62-year-old accountant, experienced Gerstmann's Syndrome after a brain tumor was removed. Although he initially struggled with writing and left-right confusion, ongoing therapy helped him relearn critical skills and return to his hobbies.

11. What tools can help manage Gerstmann's Syndrome?

Various tools and resources are available to support individuals with Gerstmann's Syndrome. Assistive technology, such as speech-to-text software and interactive math apps, can help patients overcome difficulties with writing and calculations. Visual aids, like labeled household items and directional signs, provide additional support for spatial challenges. Ergonomic writing devices and adaptive grips are also helpful for those with dysgraphia.

Lily, a young girl with developmental Gerstmann's Syndrome, used a combination of visual charts and gamified math apps to build confidence in the classroom. These tools transformed her learning experience, making previously frustrating tasks manageable and enjoyable.

12. How can families support a loved one with Gerstmann's Syndrome?

Families play a crucial role in supporting individuals with Gerstmann's Syndrome. Creating a structured and supportive environment, using visual reminders, and practicing patience are key strategies. Encouraging open communication and celebrating small victories help build confidence and resilience. Additionally, involving the patient in support groups or therapy sessions fosters a sense of empowerment.

The Johnson family transformed their approach after their son was diagnosed. They adapted their home with labeled items, sought out therapy, and joined a local support group. These steps not only improved their son's quality of life but also strengthened their family bonds.

Conclusion

Gerstmann's Syndrome presents unique challenges, but understanding its nuances can empower patients and families to navigate the condition effectively. By leveraging therapies, tools, and community support, individuals can build resilience and lead fulfilling lives. Each step forward—whether through small victories or major breakthroughs—demonstrates the strength and determination of those living with this rare condition.

16 Looking Forward

As we reach the end of this comprehensive exploration of Gerstmann's Syndrome, it becomes evident that the journey of understanding and living with this rare neurological condition is as complex as it is hopeful. From the defining tetrad of symptoms to the profound impacts on education, relationships, and daily living, this book has sought to illuminate every facet of Gerstmann's Syndrome, offering insights, strategies, and hope to patients and their families.

Reflections on the Journey

Living with Gerstmann's Syndrome, whether as a patient or a caregiver, is a journey that demands extraordinary resilience. The syndrome's unique challenges—difficulty recognizing fingers, struggles with writing and performing math, and spatial disorientation—place continuous demands on patience, adaptability, and creativity. These obstacles can sometimes feel insurmountable, but they also offer opportunities for growth, innovation, and connection. As the patient stories throughout this book have demonstrated, individuals affected by this condition often rise to meet these challenges with remarkable strength and perseverance, showcasing their ability to achieve profound growth and triumph despite the hurdles they face.

Take Emily, a young girl diagnosed with Developmental Gerstmann's Syndrome, as an example of this resilience. Her persistent struggles with math once left her feeling frustrated, isolated, and deeply discouraged, as she watched her peers excel at tasks that seemed impossible for her. However, through early intervention, a supportive educational environment, and tailored therapies that addressed her specific needs, Emily began to make measurable progress. Over time, her confidence grew alongside her abilities, and she transitioned from feeling defeated by her challenges to embracing them as stepping stones to success. Not only did she improve academically, but she also blossomed into a self-assured student who inspired her classmates and teachers alike. Her journey serves as a testament to the transformative power of understanding, targeted support, and the unwavering belief that progress is always possible with the right tools and encouragement.

Advancements in Understanding

Recent years have brought remarkable progress in understanding Gerstmann's Syndrome. Advances in neuroimaging have highlighted the critical role of the angular gyrus in integrating sensory input, motor planning, and abstract reasoning. These discoveries have not only refined diagnostic criteria but also deepened our understanding of the brain's complexities.

Yet, much remains to be explored. Why does the syndrome manifest differently in children compared to adults? How can emerging therapies, such as neuromodulation, be harnessed to address specific deficits? These questions underscore the need for ongoing research and collaboration among clinicians, educators, and families.

The Importance of Early Intervention

One of the most consistent themes throughout this book is the importance of early identification and intervention. Whether through comprehensive neuropsychological assessments or the keen observations of a teacher or parent, recognizing the signs of Gerstmann's Syndrome early opens the door to effective treatment.

Consider Liam, whose difficulties with handwriting and math were initially dismissed as developmental delays. A detailed assessment revealed the classic tetrad of symptoms, enabling his parents to seek targeted therapies. Today, Liam's confidence and academic progress reflect the profound impact of timely intervention.

Living with Gerstmann's Syndrome

For patients and families, navigating life with Gerstmann's Syndrome requires a multifaceted approach. Therapies tailored to individual needs, adaptive tools for daily tasks, and a strong support network are essential components of a fulfilling life. Chapters in this book have provided practical advice, from creating inclusive educational environments to building supportive relationships.

Maggie, a retired librarian, demonstrated how small adaptations—such as labeling household items and using visual reminders—can transform everyday life. Her resourcefulness and determination exemplify the resilience of those living with Gerstmann's Syndrome.

The Role of Advocacy and Community

No journey is undertaken alone. The stories of families like the Johnsons, who founded an advocacy group after their son's diagnosis, highlight the power of community in driving awareness and change. By uniting patients, caregivers, and professionals, advocacy groups amplify the voices of those affected by Gerstmann's Syndrome, pushing for better resources, research, and support.

Online communities have also become lifelines for many families, offering advice, empathy, and connection. Maria, a mother of three, found solace and guidance in a virtual support group, where she discovered strategies to help her son navigate his challenges.

Looking Ahead: The Future of Gerstmann's Syndrome

The future holds promise for those affected by Gerstmann's Syndrome. Research continues to uncover the neurological underpinnings of the condition, paving the way for innovative treatments. Therapies like virtual reality-based cognitive training and non-invasive brain stimulation are on the horizon, offering hope for enhanced symptom management.

Patient advocacy will remain a driving force in shaping this future. By fostering collaboration between researchers, clinicians, and families, advocacy efforts ensure that progress translates into tangible benefits for patients.

A Message of Hope

Gerstmann's Syndrome is more than a collection of symptoms—it is a testament to the brain's complexity and humanity's resilience. Each patient story shared in this book, from children like Lily and Liam to adults like Thomas and Maria, reflects the strength and determination of those navigating this condition. Their journeys inspire us to continue seeking knowledge, offering support, and building a future where every individual with Gerstmann's Syndrome can thrive.

As we look forward, let us remain committed to the principles that have guided this book: understanding, compassion, and hope. Together, we can illuminate the path ahead, ensuring that those affected by Gerstmann's Syndrome are never alone in their journey.

Appendix A: Medical Glossary.

This glossary provides definitions of key medical and neurological terms referenced throughout the book. It is designed to help readers understand complex concepts related to Gerstmann's Syndrome and associated conditions.

Acalculia

A neurological impairment characterized by difficulty in performing mathematical calculations. It is one of the hallmark symptoms of Gerstmann's Syndrome.

Agraphia

The inability to write, often resulting from damage to specific areas of the brain. In Gerstmann's Syndrome, it is linked to the angular gyrus in the parietal lobe.

Angular Gyrus

A region of the brain located in the parietal lobe, near the intersection of the temporal and occipital lobes. It plays a crucial role in integrating sensory information and is central to the symptoms of Gerstmann's Syndrome.

Aphasia

A disorder resulting in impaired language abilities, such as speaking, understanding, reading, or writing. Aphasia is distinct from Gerstmann's Syndrome but can co-occur in certain cases.

Babinski Sign

A reflex action in which the big toe bends upward while the other toes fan outward when the sole of the foot is stimulated. This response, observed in some individuals with neurological conditions, can indicate damage to the central nervous system.

Cognitive Decline

A broad term describing the deterioration of mental functions, including memory, attention, and problem-solving. It may result from various neurological conditions, including dementia and brain injuries.

Constructional Apraxia

The inability to construct or draw objects, often associated with damage to the parietal lobe. It may appear in individuals with Gerstmann's Syndrome as an additional symptom.

Developmental Gerstmann's Syndrome (DGS)

A subset of Gerstmann's Syndrome seen in children, characterized by difficulties in learning, writing, math, and spatial orientation due to atypical neurodevelopment rather than acquired brain damage.

Dyscalculia

A specific learning disability involving persistent difficulty with mathematical concepts and calculations. Dyscalculia is a key feature of both developmental and acquired forms of Gerstmann's Syndrome.

Dysgraphia

A condition affecting handwriting ability, characterized by poor letter formation, spacing, and overall legibility. In Gerstmann's Syndrome, dysgraphia results from neurological dysfunction.

Electroencephalogram (EEG)

A diagnostic test that records electrical activity in the brain using electrodes placed on the scalp. EEGs may detect abnormalities in individuals with developmental neurological conditions.

Finger Agnosia

The inability to recognize, identify, or differentiate one's own fingers. This symptom is a defining characteristic of Gerstmann's Syndrome.

Functional MRI (fMRI)

A type of magnetic resonance imaging that measures brain activity by detecting changes in blood flow. It is often used in research to study brain regions involved in specific cognitive tasks.

Graphesthesia

The ability to recognize writing on the skin by touch alone. Impairments in graphesthesia may be observed in individuals with parietal lobe dysfunctions.

Hemisphere (Brain)

The brain is divided into two hemispheres, left and right. The left hemisphere is typically dominant for language and logical reasoning, while the right hemisphere is associated with spatial and creative tasks.

Individualized Education Program (IEP)

A plan developed for children with special educational needs, outlining specific accommodations and goals to support their learning in a school setting.

Multidisciplinary Care Team

A group of healthcare professionals from various specialties who collaborate to provide comprehensive care for patients with complex conditions, such as Gerstmann's Syndrome.

Neurological Assessment

A clinical evaluation that examines brain function through cognitive, sensory, and motor tests. It helps diagnose conditions like Gerstmann's Syndrome.

Neuroplasticity

The brain's ability to reorganize itself by forming new neural connections throughout life. This capability allows the brain to adapt to injury, such as damage to the angular gyrus in Gerstmann's Syndrome, by recruiting other regions to compensate for lost functions.

Neuropsychology

A field of psychology that studies the relationship between brain function and behavior. Neuropsychological assessments are crucial in diagnosing and managing Gerstmann's Syndrome.

Parietal Lobe

A region of the brain responsible for processing sensory information, spatial reasoning, and integrating motor functions. Damage to this area can lead to symptoms of Gerstmann's Syndrome.

Rehabilitation Therapy

Therapeutic interventions designed to help individuals regain skills and adapt to physical or cognitive impairments. Common forms include occupational, physical, and speech therapy.

Right-Left Disorientation

A difficulty in distinguishing between right and left sides of the body or space. This symptom is one of the hallmark features of Gerstmann's Syndrome.

Sensory Integration

The process by which the brain organizes and interprets sensory information from the body and the environment. Impairments in sensory integration, often seen in individuals with Gerstmann's Syndrome, can affect motor skills, spatial orientation, and perception.

Stroke

A medical event caused by the interruption of blood flow to the brain, leading to tissue damage. Strokes are a common cause of acquired Gerstmann's Syndrome.

Traumatic Brain Injury (TBI)

An injury to the brain resulting from an external force, such as a blow to the head. TBI can lead to a range of neurological deficits, including the onset of Gerstmann's Syndrome in some cases.

Virtual Reality (VR) Therapy

An emerging therapeutic tool that uses immersive virtual environments to enhance cognitive and motor skills. VR therapy shows potential for managing symptoms of neurological conditions like Gerstmann's Syndrome.

Appendix B: Similar Syndromes

Gerstmann's Syndrome, with its hallmark tetrad of symptoms—finger agnosia, dysgraphia, dyscalculia, and left-right disorientation—presents unique diagnostic challenges due to its overlap with several other neurological and developmental conditions. This appendix provides an overview of syndromes and conditions that may appear similar, offering insight into the differential diagnosis process.

1. Balint's Syndrome

Balint's Syndrome is a rare neurological condition caused by bilateral parietal lobe damage. It is characterized by a triad of symptoms: optic ataxia (difficulty reaching for objects under visual guidance), ocular apraxia (difficulty controlling eye movements), and simultanagnosia (inability to perceive multiple visual elements simultaneously). While it shares some overlap with spatial and motor difficulties observed in Gerstmann's Syndrome, the visual deficits in Balint's Syndrome are distinct and not present in Gerstmann's.

2. Developmental Coordination Disorder (DCD)

Also known as dyspraxia, DCD affects fine and gross motor skills, often causing difficulties with handwriting, balance, and spatial awareness. In children, these symptoms can mimic aspects of Developmental Gerstmann's Syndrome, particularly dysgraphia and spatial challenges. However, DCD does not typically include difficulties with arithmetic or finger agnosia, distinguishing it from Gerstmann's Syndrome.

3. Apraxia

Apraxia is a motor planning disorder that impairs the ability to perform purposeful movements, despite normal muscle strength and coordination. Constructional apraxia, a specific form associated with parietal lobe lesions, can resemble the spatial difficulties seen in Gerstmann's Syndrome. However, apraxia does not encompass the full tetrad of Gerstmann's symptoms, such as dyscalculia or left-right disorientation.

4. Dyslexia

Dyslexia, a learning disorder that primarily affects reading, often overlaps with dysgraphia (difficulty with writing). While individuals with Developmental Gerstmann's Syndrome may also exhibit dyslexia, the two conditions are distinct. Dyslexia focuses on reading and language processing deficits, whereas Gerstmann's Syndrome involves additional symptoms like finger agnosia and spatial disorientation.

5. Alzheimer's Disease

Alzheimer's disease and other forms of dementia can lead to cognitive impairments, including difficulties with writing, calculation, and spatial orientation. In the early stages, these symptoms may resemble Gerstmann's Syndrome, particularly if a lesion affects the parietal lobe. However, Alzheimer's typically involves progressive memory loss and generalized cognitive decline, which are not defining features of Gerstmann's Syndrome.

6. Nonverbal Learning Disorder (NVLD)

NVLD is a developmental condition characterized by deficits in visual-spatial processing, motor coordination, and social skills. Children with NVLD may exhibit challenges similar to those with Developmental Gerstmann's Syndrome, including left-right disorientation and difficulty with mathematics. However,

NVLD does not include finger agnosia, distinguishing it from Gerstmann's Syndrome.

7. Acalculia

Acalculia, or acquired difficulty with mathematical tasks, is often a symptom of broader neurological damage, including parietal lobe lesions. While it is a component of Gerstmann's Syndrome, acalculia can also occur in isolation or alongside other conditions, such as aphasia or traumatic brain injury.

8. Stroke

Strokes affecting the parietal lobe may result in symptoms overlapping with Gerstmann's Syndrome. However, stroke presentations are highly variable and often accompanied by additional motor, sensory, or language deficits, depending on the location and extent of the damage. A detailed neurological assessment is necessary to differentiate between stroke-related impairments and Gerstmann's Syndrome.

9. Right-Left Disorientation Syndrome

Right-left disorientation, a symptom of Gerstmann's Syndrome, can also appear in isolation or as part of other neurological conditions, such as multiple sclerosis or traumatic brain injury. The presence of this symptom alone is insufficient for a Gerstmann's diagnosis, emphasizing the need to identify the full tetrad.

10. Finger Agnosia

Finger agnosia, or difficulty identifying one's own fingers, is a hallmark of Gerstmann's Syndrome but can also occur in isolation due to localized parietal damage. Conditions like traumatic brain injury or specific neurodevelopmental disorders may feature finger agnosia without the broader context of Gerstmann's Syndrome.

11. Constructional Apraxia

This disorder involves difficulty constructing or drawing objects, often due to parietal lobe damage. While constructional apraxia may accompany Gerstmann's Syndrome, it is not part of the syndrome's defining tetrad and may arise independently.

12. Autism Spectrum Disorder (ASD)

Children with autism spectrum disorder may exhibit motor coordination challenges, spatial disorientation, or difficulties with writing. However, the core social communication deficits and repetitive behaviors characteristic of ASD help distinguish it from Developmental Gerstmann's Syndrome.

13. Posterior Cortical Atrophy (PCA)

A rare neurodegenerative condition often associated with Alzheimer's disease, PCA affects the parietal and occipital lobes, leading to visual and spatial impairments. While it shares features with Gerstmann's Syndrome, PCA is progressive and typically includes pronounced visual deficits.

Appendix C: Resources

This appendix lists trusted organizations, websites, and support groups to help individuals with Gerstmann's Syndrome and their families access reliable information, connect with others, and find specialized care. Whenever possible, contact information, including canonical URLs and phone numbers, has been included for easy access.

1. National Institute of Neurological Disorders and Stroke (NINDS)

The NINDS provides authoritative information on neurological conditions, including Gerstmann's Syndrome. Their website includes research updates, treatment options, and links to clinical trials.

- **Website**: https://www.ninds.nih.gov
- **Phone**: +1-800-352-9424
- **Email**: braininfo@ninds.nih.gov

2. American Academy of Neurology (AAN)

The AAN connects patients with neurologists specializing in conditions like Gerstmann's Syndrome. Their site includes a directory to find certified providers and resources for understanding neurological disorders.

- **Website**: https://www.aan.com
- **Phone**: +1-612-928-6000

3. Child Neurology Foundation (CNF)

For families navigating developmental forms of Gerstmann's Syndrome, the CNF offers resources tailored to children, including support networks, webinars, and educational materials.

- **Website**: https://www.childneurologyfoundation.org
- **Phone**: +1-612-928-6325
- **Email**: info@childneurologyfoundation.org

4. Brain & Behavior Research Foundation

This organization funds research into brain disorders and provides updates on breakthroughs in neuroscience that may impact conditions like Gerstmann's Syndrome.

- **Website**: https://www.bbrfoundation.org
- **Phone**: +1-646-681-4888
- **Email**: info@bbrfoundation.org

5. National Organization for Rare Disorders (NORD)

NORD offers support and resources for individuals with rare conditions, including Gerstmann's Syndrome. Their database includes patient stories, research links, and advocacy opportunities.

- **Website**: https://rarediseases.org
- **Phone**: +1-800-999-6673
- **Email**: orphan@rarediseases.org

6. Dyscalculia Network

A specialized resource for individuals struggling with mathematical challenges, including dyscalculia, which is a hallmark feature of Gerstmann's Syndrome. The network offers teaching strategies and support tools.

- **Website**: https://www.dyscalculianetwork.com
- **Email**: info@dyscalculianetwork.com

7. Learning Disabilities Association of America (LDA)

The LDA provides educational resources and advocacy for individuals with learning disabilities, including developmental Gerstmann's Syndrome. Their tools support parents, educators, and caregivers.

- **Website**: https://www.ldaamerica.org
- **Phone**: +1-412-341-1515
- **Email**: info@ldaamerica.org

8. Neuropsychology Central

An online hub for neuropsychologists and patients seeking insights into brain-behavior relationships. This site includes directories to find specialists and articles on conditions like Gerstmann's Syndrome.

- **Website**: https://www.neuropsychologycentral.com

9. American Occupational Therapy Association (AOTA)

Occupational therapists play a key role in helping individuals with Gerstmann's Syndrome adapt to daily challenges. The AOTA offers resources for finding specialists and understanding occupational therapy's benefits.

- **Website**: https://www.aota.org
- **Phone**: +1-301-652-6611
- **Email**: feedback@aota.org

10. RareConnect

A platform connecting patients with rare conditions, including Gerstmann's Syndrome. RareConnect facilitates patient discussions and provides a space for sharing experiences and advice.

- **Website**: https://www.rareconnect.org

11. Understood.org

This site offers tools and resources for parents of children with learning disabilities. Their articles and community forums include practical advice for managing conditions like developmental Gerstmann's Syndrome.

- **Website**: https://www.understood.org

12. Mayo Clinic

The Mayo Clinic's website provides reliable, easy-to-understand information on Gerstmann's Syndrome, including symptoms, diagnostic procedures, and treatment options.

- **Website**: https://www.mayoclinic.org

13. Facebook Support Groups

Several Facebook groups connect individuals and families affected by Gerstmann's Syndrome. These groups foster community support and allow members to share experiences and coping strategies.

- **Search on Facebook:** Use keywords like "Gerstmann's Syndrome Support Group" to find active communities.

How to Use These Resources

- **Start with Medical Organizations**: For accurate and research-based information, prioritize resources like NINDS, AAN, and NORD.

- **Join Support Networks**: Online platforms such as RareConnect and Facebook support groups offer a sense of community and shared experiences.

- **Seek Professional Guidance**: Use directories provided by organizations like AOTA and AAN to find specialists familiar with Gerstmann's Syndrome.

By leveraging these resources, individuals with Gerstmann's Syndrome and their families can find the guidance, support, and community needed to navigate life with this condition effectively.

Disclaimer

This book is here to provide helpful information and insights, but it's not meant to replace professional medical advice, diagnosis, or treatment. We encourage you to talk to a qualified healthcare provider if you have questions or concerns about your health or medical care. While we've done our best to include accurate information, this book is intended as a general guide, and we can't guarantee every detail. For specific medical advice or guidance, please reach out to your doctor or healthcare team.

ABOUT THE AUTHOR

Steph White is an accomplished health science writer with over 30 years of experience, dedicated to transforming complex medical information into clear, actionable insights. With an undergraduate degree in Health Sciences and two master's degrees, she brings a deep understanding of medical topics to her work, making it accessible to readers from all walks of life. Her passion for health education is not only rooted in her professional background but also in her personal journey living with a rare disease. This firsthand experience has shaped her empathetic approach, enabling her to connect with patients and families navigating the uncertainties of rare diagnoses.

Throughout her career, Steph has worked on numerous projects aimed at educating patients, caregivers, and healthcare providers, earning a reputation for technical accuracy and relatable language. Her writing bridges the gap between medical science and everyday understanding, reflecting her commitment to empowering individuals with knowledge. Steph's unique blend of expertise and compassion shines through in her work, inspiring hope and fostering understanding among her readers.

About This Guide

The Gerstmann's Syndrome Sourcebook is your essential companion for understanding and managing this rare and complex neurological condition. Written by Steph White, a health science writer with over 30 years of experience, this guide blends technical accuracy with deep compassion to provide patients, families, and caregivers with the knowledge they need to navigate life with Gerstmann's Syndrome.

In this comprehensive resource, you'll find:

- Clear explanations of the hallmark symptoms, including finger agnosia, dysgraphia, dyscalculia, and left-right disorientation.
- Insightful explorations of the neurological causes, risk factors, and diagnostic processes.
- Practical strategies for daily living, educational success, and building supportive relationships.
- Stories of resilience and triumph from individuals and families living with the condition.

Steph White brings a unique perspective to this work—not only as an expert writer with degrees in Health Sciences but also as someone living with a rare disease herself. Her personal journey fuels her commitment to making health information accessible and actionable for all.

Whether you're newly diagnosed, supporting a loved one, or seeking to deepen your understanding, *The Gerstmann's Syndrome Sourcebook* is an empowering, compassionate guide to navigating the complexities of this condition with confidence and hope.

www.ingramcontent.com/pod-product-compliance
Lightning Source LLC
Chambersburg PA
CBHW071059240526
45471CB00016B/2166